YOU DON'T HAVE
CANCE

YOU DON'T HAVE TO DIE
FROM CANCER

Taking Active Charge

by

Dr Abraham Khazam

HILL OF CONTENT

Melbourne

To Sharon

First published in Australia 1996
by Hill of Content Publishing
86 Bourke Street
Melbourne 3000

© Copyright Dr Abraham Khazam 1996

Typeset by Figment Productions Pty Ltd, Fitzroy, Victoria
Printed by Australian Print Group

National Library of Australia
Cataloguing-in-publication data
Khazam, Abraham, 1931–
    You don't have to die from cancer: taking active charge.

    Bibliography.
    ISBN 0 85572 266 5
    1. Cancer – Popular works. 2. Cancer – Psychological aspects.
    3. Cancer – Treatment. I. Title

616.994

CONTENTS

CONTENTS (continued)

PART FOUR: HEALING

INTRODUCTION

This book was written primarily for the person who has cancer, whether or not s/he decides to become a patient and to undergo medical treatment. I also hope that it may be useful to those who are able to give support to this person, such as doctors, nursing staff, relatives, and friends. If you have cancer, you may need support in your task to become bodily and emotionally fit enough to cope with the emotional and physical problems of this disorder: don't hesitate to ask for help.

A positive attitude among your immediate social circle may be as beneficial as a negative one can be harmful.

Our concern is not how cancer cells are born from our normal cells, but how it is that these cells are allowed to stay and grow, and what stops the body from getting rid of them, as it does generally with such invasions. We shall also pass by the question of the possible importance of diet and environment, and concentrate on the emotional side of having cancer.

If we are to fight an enemy, we must know this enemy, so that we know what we can and cannot do about it. We must identify our opponent, to avoid thinking of it as some mysterious agent that is too powerful for our efforts. We will do this and find that cancer is nothing more mysterious than a special kind of infection. Knowing this, we are better prepared to cope with it. Not only must we know our enemy, and assess its strength, we must also know ourselves, and estimate our own power; we can do this through visualisation, and this book will show you how it should be performed.

We focus on what happens further to this infection after the initial invasion of our organism, and we consider how we can stop this infection from growing and spreading, and how we may recover from it. We turn our attention to the defensive and healing functions of the human organism in health, and how it may be affected by emotional stress. We examine the nature of biological cancer as an infection, and see what this means for healing and defence in general.

The treatment of cancer (oncotherapy) with drugs and radiation should not be regarded as a small matter, because it is just as traumatic as any major surgical operation. We should make ourselves ready for it, and try to become as fit as possible for coping with this physical cancer treatment. Preparing patients for any major operation should not be limited to preparing the body for it, which is still too much the only routine in many hospitals. The personal-emotional dimension of the patient is almost neglected in this traditional routine.

Just as a full blood count is needed to make sure that the blood spectrum is normal before the operation, an attempt should be made to lighten the considerable emotional burden of the patient. As a patient we are not only a compliant body; we are a person, an emotionally sensitive and aware organism, who carries the load of worries that comes with any operation.

We are inevitably involved in our own healing, whether or not this fact is being recognised; and if we don't take some care to make this involvement a positive contribution to healing, then by default it becomes counterproductive.

Unless the person of the patient (not just the body) is taken into consideration, it may not be reasonable to expect sound healing to take place after any major operation with scalpel, radiation or drug. It is universally recognised medical experience that stress results in poor defence and healing; yet not enough is done about this. The personal side of illness is ignored in the preoccupation with advanced medical techniques.

If the person, the total organism, who is about to undergo any kind of medical treatment is emotionally prepared, it will make a significant difference; this is the experience of psychosomatic medicine. There are surgeons and oncologists who are beginning to apply this in their work with patients.

The patient is a complete human organism, and cannot afford to ignore her (or his) own responsibility in the proper preparation for healing. I emphasise in this book that this person must learn to take active charge of the whole process, and I indicate how it is to be achieved. A ground rule of psychosomatic medicine is that a patient must take active charge of her/his own illness and welfare, because healing is not merely a body routine; the total organism is in charge of it.

R. Magnus, an eminent neurophysiologist, wrote an influential book about his investigations into the way cats right themselves during a fall. He came to this conclusion: it is not the cat's nervous system that directs this process of landing on its feet, but it is the organism itself that determines the right processes in its nervous system. (R. Magnus, quoted by F. J. J. Buytendijk, *Algemene theorie der menselijke houding en beweging*, pages 186, 258, 401). What happens inside the nervous system, said Buytendijk (same book, page 401), only mirrors the interaction between an organism and its world.

This is true because the body is part of the total organism, and the nervous system is part of this body. It is always the total that determines the part, and never the part that guides the total. It is the human being who thinks, said E. Straus, and not his brain (*Vom Sinn der Sinne*, page 112). That total human being whom we know as the mind or as the person, we may say, makes use of the body for its regular routines. The body is only the formed part of the mind. The mind, said the French philosopher Henri Bergson, exceeds the brain, and is larger than the body. Our life is part routine, and part change and novelty. It is for the sake of that automatic, habitual, routine in our interaction with the world we live in, that we (the mind) need a body.

Professors Prick and van de Loo of the Netherlands examined patients with rheumatoid arthritis, and found that personality and this disease are here closely bound up; signs of psychological changes were found earlier than the outbreak of body symptoms (K. M. van de Loo, *Psychosomatiek*, page 43). Professors Prick, Groen, and Bastiaans (all important names in psychosomatic medicine), found this to be true also for multiple sclerosis (page 44).

A passive patient is a helpless person, and helpless is something no modern patient can afford to be. This person will struggle to recover, because helplessness means failure. It indicates that we can't cope, that we have either given up trying to cope or, worse, we haven't even begun to try it and we are beaten before we start.

Our 'body', as only a part of our total existence, cannot be trusted to look after itself in any serious disease, because by becoming ill, this body already indicates that it is in a state of failure. Our mind, being bigger and better than the body, must guide it, and support it in healing.

The body is only the sum of the fixed routines of the complete organism that we call the mind. Healing is not a routine of the body, it is the task of the entire organism, of the mind.

In any supportive interaction with cancer patients there are certain questions that keep coming up, questions that relate to hope and despair, to what is truth and what false hope, to the precise meaning of statistical data, and many more. These are questions that come with all serious illnesses, and they have been discussed to some extent in excellent books, such as Simonton and Creighton's *Getting Well Again* (also known as 'the cancer patient's bible') and *Love, Medicine and Miracles*, by Bernie Siegel.

We need to go deeper into these questions, however, because of their great importance for the well-being of those who suffer from the cancer, as well as that of their supporting relatives and friends. Proper support by this social circle is very important for the general well-being of the cancer patient, as we shall see; and the people around the patient should also understand the emotional nature of the situation.

Such emotionally charged questions can be asked, and answered, on two different levels, and this must be clearly understood. We may ask a question that could, to the untrained ear, sound like a normal request for objective information, but that is a different question on our emotional level. An objective answer to such a highly primed question may not even be heard as such while it is understood on the emotional level in the form of a paralysing 'kick in the stomach', a 'squeezing fist around the heart' or in a sense of utter desolation: 'Oh God I'm finished!'

Telling the objective truth to someone in emotional disarray is about as useful for healing as saying it in an unfamiliar foreign language: it won't be received as an objective truth. The rational mind, said Dr Heyer in his book on psychotherapy (*Praktische Seelenheilkunde*, page 18), is illiterate when it comes to emotional affairs, and this means that 'telling it as it is' is merely information for the rational mind that the emotional mind cannot digest. We shall see that our emotional mind is capable of understanding objective information only if it is relatively at ease; if not, then it is in no condition to understand any rational information. It simply cannot hear this as it is; if it is able to listen, it hears something else, and this different message may cause much unnecessary damage.

The reader may notice that some issues in this book seem to be repeated in different chapters; this is done deliberately for two good reasons. The first is that such important points will be remembered better, and the second reason for the repetition is this: it will show that we can come to these central issues from a number of different directions.

This intersection of different directions tells us that we are keeping to the right track in our reasoning. If all roads lead to Rome, as the saying goes, then these different directions become so many arrows that point to it as a fact. We then have the satisfaction that it all comes together.

I have made a reasonable attempt to go through the literature that is available to me, to ensure as much as possible that I give credit where it is due. It is impossible to read all that there is on this and related subjects. I therefore freely offer my apologies to those that I may have overlooked, and I would appreciate being notified of corrections that should be made.

The proper use of relaxation and visualisation in healing is of course as old as hypnosis, and it has been applied to emotional healing since the early part of this century.

Systematic body relaxation began with Jacobson in the US (*Progressive Relaxation*), and Schultz in Germany (*Autogenic Training*). Having learned the technique of Autogenic Training while I was studying medicine in Holland in 1959, and having practised it ever since, I naturally prefer it as the better method; it goes beyond mere systematic muscle relaxation. Using autogenic training we learn to influence our internal and involuntary functions, and to do it by an intense passive concentration on visualised functions. For many reasons, autogenic training may well be said to be the father of biofeedback.

VIEWPOINT AND SOME STRATEGIES

Written by a general practitioner with considerable experience in psychiatry and a deep interest in psychosomatic medicine, this book will show cancer patients mostly as seen from general practice: that is, the emotional side of having cancer.

The book will not necessarily reflect the view of the oncologist, because specialist and general practitioner may see the 'same' patient in two different situations. Each viewpoint will show the patient in a somewhat different light, because the focus of their interest and treatment is different.

The immediate reason for writing this book is the need to call attention to the important fact that there is more to 'having cancer' than the mere presence of biological cancer tissue in the body. In concentrating on the problems of the biological cancer, we seem to have overlooked two serious emotional complications that have gone mostly unrecognised or unnoticed in the clamour over the biological cancer.

These are both serious emotional illnesses that can and should be prevented. If they are already present, then they must be recognised and treated with urgency: they represent two forms of demoralisation that come at different times, and are motivated by different emotions.

The presence of such demoralisation has been noted, of course, but usually merely waved away as an 'understandable reaction' to having cancer. These demoralisation syndromes are anything but that, however; they are emotional disorders in their own right, and represent an abnormal reaction to having cancer. They are psychological cancers that have wormed their way into the darker regions of the emotional mind, where they proceed with their destructive work.

There are two such emotional disorders and they are both forms of demoralisation:

1 *Voodoo death.* Certain vulnerable personalities develop a malignant belief in the myth that one must inevitably die from cancer: this is a severe emotional disorder that may lead to a

psychogenic death. This illness occurs soon after the diagnosis, and patients die unnecessarily, long before the cancer may end their life. The term psychogenic means stemming from the (emotional) mind, and here refers to a death by self-destruction which is based on a wrong conviction that one must die: it is also known as a voodoo or bone-pointing death.

This 'cancer patient' presents with an early demoralisation syndrome that, unless treated, may lead to an unnecessary and premature psychogenic death. This illness is a preventable and treatable psychosis that is motivated by an almost delusional certainty of being slated to die. These persons do not fight, they give up from the very beginning what they perceive as a hopeless condition. Fighting is not even an option to them.

2 *Battle fatigue.* The second form of emotional illness is a battle fatigue syndrome that occurs later: a coping failure at the end of a long struggle. This is a battle against the cancer itself, against the gnawing daily uncertainty of the fight, against the indignities of cancer therapy and, finally, against the embarrassment and guilt of being an inconvenience or burden to the family. This family has by now, usually become somewhat less tolerant of the continuing illness.

Such battle weariness occurs in the fighter personality, who does not give up from the start, but who fights what she or he now perceives, in the end, as a losing fight. These people finally give up the fight, feeling worn out from trying; death has become a real and even acceptable option.

In this book, the question of whether cancer can be caused by stress is only a side issue; we concentrate instead on another aspect of cancer that needs special attention, because it may lead to a totally unnecessary early death. It is preventable, and has nothing to do with the growth of the biological cancer itself, it is an emotional cancer that works like a hypnotic instruction to die soon. It is, as we shall see, a psychogenic death that is similar to a voodoo death.

The late demoralisation of the fighting spirit of the patient, which is due to battle fatigue, will also need to be looked at.

We shall discuss the nature of this psychological cancer and its neutralisation. Another topic that is examined is the nature of the biological cancer as an infection, and what this means for healing in general.

We must also focus on the principles of healing; this is the function of becoming whole again: healing, hale, health, and whole, are related concepts. In medicine we take it for granted that people heal; how such natural healing takes place is usually only studied in its anatomical-physiological form, which does not include the mind or personality of the patient.

If the patient does not heal, according to this view, then it is the fault of the body, and just bad luck if this happens. How well patients are motivated to heal is traditionally left to themselves and to chance, and it is unfortunate that this has not been sufficiently recognised outside the field of psychosomatic medicine. Traditional medicine tries to prevent disease and death by treatment, but does not teach healing, and this must change.

It is an ancient tradition that soldiers who go into battle have first to be well-motivated and well-nourished; an army, said Napoleon, travels on its stomach. Soldiers are mentally and physically trained for battle, so that they are fighting fit and well-motivated, their morale high.

Professional athletes (and other public performers) often employ sport psychologists to help them build up their self-confidence, and to boost their motivation to win. They rehearse a perfect performance in their mind while they are in a state of relaxation, and they achieve this by means of visualisation techniques. Such athletes enter competition with high expectations and a determination to do their utmost to win.

If this motivation is so important for soldiers and athletes and public performers of any kind, why is it not important that patients who must undergo surgery, or fight some disease, should be similarly fighting fit, with high morale and sense of self-worth, before the big battle for recovery and health? Is this not a performance worthy of attention? Don't we fight a similar battle every time we suffer from an infection or trauma, and don't we struggle to recover from operations? Every patient deserves – and thus should have – such training in the techniques of healing and recovery.

Performance training is a method that has proven itself in war, in hypnosis, in sport, and lately even in business. Why is it still not systematically introduced in medicine to boost healing?

Is medicine suffering from a neurosis that makes it cling to outdated traditions, and closed to such modern approaches to healing? In medical tradition the patient is a passive element in the technical dialogue between diseased body and doctor, so that his or her personal feelings count for little. The personality of the patient is usually barely tolerated, and the ideal patient is the one under anaesthesia.

It is no accident that psychology was a latecomer in medicine, and that it is still too often viewed with suspicion: 'Hmm, all that modern nonsense. Imagine taking an active role in your own healing, instead of properly leaving it to surgeons and drugs; what next, I wonder?'

From their conservative point of view, such people have viewed the psychological sciences with suspicion, because they have been unable to imagine that the person has some input in her or his own illness and recovery. Psychosomatic medicine has irrevocably introduced the patient as an actively involved person into illness and healing.

The patient must no longer remain a passive factor in his or her own healing, because medicine cannot, and should not, do without this person's competent involvement in healing. The active participation of the patient is of vital importance in healing. This is the fundamental rule of psychosomatic medicine.

A growing number of patients now demand a more total psychosomatic approach to their problems. The modern patient is no longer satisfied to remain a passive onlooker in her or his own recovery, and wants and needs to be taught to heal.

Reinhold Niebuhr (quoted in Spiegel H., and Spiegel D.: *Trances and Treatment*, page 175) offered this prayer: 'Give me the strength to change that which can be changed, the courage to accept that which cannot be changed, and the wisdom to tell one from the other.' This fine sentence could serve as the motto for this book.

The chapters that follow have been organised into three parts:

Part one describes the voodoo and battle fatigue states; Part two explains, in easy terms, the biology of cancer as an infection, and the regulation of defence and healing systems; Part three discusses the psychology of cancer and stress; Part four is dedicated to the nature and meaning of healing and its techniques, for both the psychological and biological cancers.

The final chapter gives a broader view on some topics for those readers who want more background.

Part One

The Diagnosis

Chapter One

THE CANCER PATIENT

This is not a book about alternative medicine, nor is it a text on the physical treatment of cancer, about surgery and oncology. It is a book about the cancer patient. Who is this patient? It is that emotional person who has been diagnosed as having cancer somewhere in the body, and who is now in a state of emotional crisis.

We take a good look at this emotional crisis in the life of the typical cancer patient, to see what this state of crisis really means, and how we should deal with it. This particular emotional crisis is not like any other emotional crisis situation in our life, because it has specific features that may hamper healing and recovery, and even promote the growth of the cancer, unless we do something about it.

There are emotional (psychological) problems that may lead to a premature and totally unnecessary death, unless we become aware of their existence, and know that we can avoid them.

PATIENT AND DOCTOR

Modern technological medicine is often so preoccupied with the physical treatment of the cancer by surgery, chemotherapy, and radiotherapy, that the treatment of the person suffering from this cancer is often overlooked, or worse, not regarded as an essential part of treatment.

Oncology focuses mainly on the biological cancer in the body, and often looks past the patient, past the person who suffers from the cancer. Books on oncology usually contain a chapter on the emotional difficulties facing cancer patients, but do not go deeply enough into the nature of this emotional crisis.

The cancer patient, who is an emotional person in crisis, in despair, is all too often neglected. The crisis is dismissed as a natural reaction to having cancer. But is it so normal?

The main reason for this neglect is, of course, that cancer is still regarded as an entirely biological problem, a disorder of the body that could not have much to do with the emotional state of mind of the patient.

The suffering of the patient is regarded as being secondary to having cancer, in the same way as the emotional problems that come with a broken leg are not usually the concern of the orthopaedic specialist. These problems have little to do with bone healing. (At least, this seemed true according to the older medical tradition.)

Oncologists may be sympathetic about emotional difficulties of their patients, of course, but emotional problems are not part of their speciality and they may feel that these are not their business. They may refer patients to appropriate psychiatrists or psychologists, if they become aware of the problem.

Oncology is about treating cancer, but not the cancer patient. Treating the cancer patient is part of psychosomatic medicine. Evidence is slowly but surely mounting that emotional problems associated with having cancer are not just a result of finding the cancer in the body. There is growing evidence that:

(a) The emotional mind may be deeply involved with the presence of growing cancer in the body, and we shall discuss this in the second part of this book.

(b) The course of cancer treatment may be strongly influenced by the motivational state (emotional mindset) of the patient, that person suffering from the cancer.

Let us put this second point more clearly: what happens to the cancer patient in the early months after the diagnosis has been made may depend almost entirely on his or her emotional mindset. A wrong mind-set may lead to more trouble, while a positive one is geared to recovery. Later in the course of the treatment, the patient becomes threatened by battle fatigue, and may develop a readiness to give up the fight and succumb to the illness.

A wrong mindset may lead to a totally unnecessary death, one that may be avoided with a better, positive, attitude. We examine this wrong mindset, and work out how it must be changed.

You, the cancer patient, can never stay neutral in this battle against cancer. Make it your fight. If you don't take up this contest against it, you may help it along by being passive. Your mind may be filled with wrong ideas about cancer, myths that you believe in, and take for granted.

The person with cancer we shall call *the typical cancer patient*, is the individual who has wrong and harmful notions in her or his emotional mind about 'cancer'.

There is more to cancer treatment than the treatment of the cancer. There is a *biological cancer* which the oncologist has specialised in, but there is also a *psychological cancer* which is a cancer in the emotional mind of the patient. This also requires urgent treatment.

The typical cancer patient is in a state of emotional disarray and, because of this, highly vulnerable to what people say and do around him or her. What some specialists could be more aware of, is just how frightened cancer patients become of their rational and clinical attitude towards them, at a time when they desperately need some emotional support.

In the same detached way that a bone specialist talks to a patient about a broken bone, the oncologist may discuss the state of the cancer with the hapless patient – without being clearly aware of the enormous difference.

For the doctor what are neutral words, may mean something else to the patient whose life is at stake, and who only hears what is said in terms of living longer or dying sooner.

The objective attitude that specialists often adopt towards their patients is a problem in itself. This attitude is partly the result of the legal requirement to hide nothing from their patient. But this may often become an excuse for ignoring the patient's emotional state of mind. Sometimes doctors may make casual and thoughtless technical comments to patients as if the patients were suffering from some merely annoying problem. Even trained doctors and nurses cannot be objective about this if they themselves are the patient. Who can remain truly objective if one's own life is at stake?

Cancer patients are very frightened people, even if they don't always show it. These are human beings in despair who tend to hang on the words of their doctors, and scrutinise every word they utter and every gesture they make, hoping for a good word, and fearing a bad one.

Cancer patients are emotional beings who have strong feelings about their condition, and who can be highly sensitive to the words and gestures of their doctors and other people in their environment.

Cancer patients anxiously watch their doctors, and absorb what they say very deeply. Doctors must know this, and choose their words carefully, not carelessly. A thoughtless comment, even a frown, expressed quite unintentionally, can mean long days of suffering. Such words and gestures are usually interpreted by emotionally charged patients in ways that have generally little to do with their intended objective meaning.

This difference is not to be wondered at, when we realise that cancer patients can often see and hear what doctors say and do with highly emotional eyes and ears: it is their life that is being discussed.

Doctor and patient talk a different language. The doctor gives a biological version of test-results. The patient hears a completely different version, and this is an emotional version that is more like a sentencing, more like a bad dream than a lesson in biology.

Many patients come to fear the consistently negative attitude that some doctors, often unwittingly, have: the doctors feel that they must be frank and not give false hope, and that they must always suspect the worst so that they tend to predict the worst possible outcome. In many cases doctors are forced to do so by the spectre of legal complications if they don't. Sparing the patient may invite legal trouble.

So every time the patient reports some pain or discomfort to the oncologist, it is usually pessimistically received as an indication of worsening unless proved otherwise. This is a sound clinical rule for a doctor to follow, because it will prevent making mistakes, but for a frightened patient it is a disaster, another horrible pointer to the expected and feared end.

Specialists may of course also be motivated by what they think of as being realistic; if so, then they have a most peculiar sense of realism. We shall examine later what being realistic means in practice.

Not all specialists are so rigidly cautious or indifferent and there are many highly sympathetic oncologists, particularly female oncologists, who can be considerably more sensitive to this issue. They are usually far more aware of their powerful status (in the emotional mind of the patient) as givers or takers of hope.

The rational mind of the patient is often a helpless spectator that remains unheard in this highly charged relationship of an emotionally vulnerable and dependent patient to the doctor. A male doctor is less likely to have an intuitively protective nature, and may remain unaware of this emotional dependency of the patient, or be unwilling to enter it.

Many patients become fearful of (what they see as) a negative attitude in their oncologist or, at least, what they experience as an attitude that is not supportive enough, and sometimes downright discouraging. The oncologist is legally bound to tell the patient the whole truth and is often careful to avoid wishful thinking, in order to remain as clinically objective as possible. But the patient suffers, and we shall see that this experience is not just hurtful or annoying. It can be potentially harmful because it amounts to what could be called a bone-pointing attitude.

There is no need to put up with this indifferent attitude from your doctor. Take charge of yourself, and find yourself a more sensitive person.

THE EMOTIONAL MIND AND CANCER

What patients themselves can contribute to their own welfare is often of vital (and always of considerable) importance in the fight against cancer. The attitude of the patient is the factor that can make all the difference, as our medical experiences with tuberculosis, a monster of the recent past, have proved. William Osler, a famous American physician, said that what happens to a patient with tuberculosis depends more on what he has in his mind than what is in his chest (quoted in F. Dunbar, Emotions and bodily changes, page li). And we may perhaps say the same about cancer.

Cancer as a psychosomatic problem is now a topic in some modern textbooks of psychiatry, and a large amount of literature is available on the deep involvement of the emotional mind in the cancer problem.

Flanders Dunbar, who wrote one of the most important earlier books on psychosomatic medicine, remarked that it does not matter whether the mind or the body is the primary seat of the disorder, in either case it is the patient who must be treated first, then the disease itself, and only in last place the symptom (F. Dunbar, same book, same page).

This means that the patient's emotional mind plays a central role in becoming sick, and in healing from the sickness. It also means that the person, with his or her emotional mind, is so deeply involved in the illness, that she or he must no longer be bypassed in the primary treatment of this illness.

What modern psychosomatic medicine teaches, is that the person is always actively involved in her or his illness, and that means that this person is either working for the illness, or against it and for healing, but that he or she can never be neutral in this affair. This is not merely an intellectual cooperation, but an involvement on the emotional level, and using powerful emotional logic. The patient must always become actively and positively involved in her or his own healing.

One can very easily get lost in the jungle of opinions and investigations regarding the role of the cancer patient in the cancer problem. Let us therefore simplify this for a more effective understanding: there are two entirely different cancers involved in every case of 'cancer':

(a) There is the biological cancer, the abnormal cell-tissue;

(b) There is also the psychological cancer. This is the cancer that preys on the emotional mind, and this is the cancer that may become quite dangerous to the patient after the biological cancer has been diagnosed.

You, the cancer patient, have this vital job to do: get rid of the psychological cancer whatever else happens. This alone will increase your chances of recovery considerably. In addition, it now makes you free to fight: to assist mother nature in the battle against the biological cancer. After all, it is in her interest that you recover; she works hard for your healing.

This is why every cancer patient must make a decision. If you resign yourself to 'having cancer' as a passive patient, you promote it by default with a wrong mental attitude that discourages healing and recovery. You must choose. If you don't work against the cancer you work for it.

The earlier experiences with the fight against tuberculosis seem to have already been forgotten; they showed that the emotional and physical well-being of the patient was vitally important for their recovery from the illness, and that it was at least as important as the physical form of treatment.

There is the local disease, cancer or tuberculosis, and there is also the patient who is suffering from this local disorder, and from the emotional crisis that these bodily diseases bring with them. There are therefore two dis-orders that need to be treated.

That this patient must become involved in the treatment in an active role, and not remain a passive carrier of the illness and that this patient must even take the driver's seat in her or his own treatment, is the most important insight of modern psychosomatic medicine. And this applies to cancer.

Don't be a passive patient, but take charge: it is your own life, and you must decide what happens to it. You have a say in what happens to you, so don't just passively and helplessly submit yourself to treatment by others.

The medical evidence is undeniable: the positive attitude of taking charge and avoiding passive suffering, is crucially important in the fight against both cancers, and that cannot be postponed or avoided. The hope for improvement is not an idle hope, it is not an illusion, but a realistic expectation.

This book, then, aims to complement the physical treatment of cancer: it is addressed to the cancer patient, the person who must stop being a hopeless and helpless patient without fight, and who must now take charge and begin the battle for health.

It is my hope that this book may also be useful for medical and supporting staff in their approach to the person with cancer.

We must examine the powerful emotional forces that influence our well-being, forces that can heal, but that can also create disorder in our system. These factors have been identified but not yet gathered into a workable system, and by workable system we mean a practical method that tells us what to do and how to do it. This is our task in this book: to present the cancer patient with this method that puts all this scattered information in one useful perspective.

These emotional factors can be separated into two convenient and obvious groups:

(a) The positive emotional factors that, taken together, make up the positive mindset that promotes healing.

(b) The wrong, negative, emotional factors that, together, form the wrong mindset that works against healing. This mindset is always found in a special situation, and we shall discuss this later as *entrapment*.

The cancer patient is the person who has been told that she or he has cancer, and is in an emotional crisis. After days, weeks, spent in anxious waiting for the diagnosis of the suspected problem, it is now definite: 'I'm sorry to say that you have cancer.' The life that went on so routinely before the diagnosis, now comes to a sudden halt.

All previous values and preoccupations now seem trivial against such terrible news, at least, until the shock wears off somewhat. It is now time to take oneself in hand, and to take stock of the quality of the life that went on before. It is also time to take stock of what must happen now.

We shall explore this scenario in the next chapter. What happens in the specialist's rooms is important for a better understanding of the right mental attitude.

Chapter Two

THE DIAGNOSIS AND ITS CONSEQUENCES

Let us follow a typical cancer patient, and look at what can happen to someone who has been found to have cancer. We shall explain that this person is now suffering from two 'cancers'. The first is located in the person's body and consists of abnormal cell tissue; this is a biological cancer.

A second 'cancer' exists in the patient's mind as a negative mental set, as a psychological cancer that eats at her or him. This emotional cancer may, in the first few months after the diagnosis, be even more malignant and dangerous than the one in the body.

This typical cancer patient is usually, but not always, the so called type C (C for cancer) or cancer-prone personality. The responsible stress-factor is said to be an enduring period of severe stress (bereavement, depression from other causes) some time before the onset of the cancer. The meeting between a cancer-prone personality and a stress situation is thought to promote the growth of cancer.

THE NATURE OF CANCER

The story of cancer may be conveniently separated into two phases:

(a) The birth of the cancer cell as a biological accident.

(b) What happens to the cancer cell after birth, in the further development of the cancer into a clinically detectable cancer. The time between the birth and diagnosis of the cancer is a silent period, in which the cancer is allowed to grow until it is detected.

The general well-being of the organism as a whole, may play an important part during this phase. It may resist or promote the growth of the cancer. General well-being also includes the condition of the emotional mind: a mind being well or in a state of stress.

There is no single cause of cancer, and we know that a variety of factors may be responsible: heredity, viruses, chemicals, radiation, and so on. These are involved in the birth of the cancer cells, and may also play a role in its further growth. Enduring emotional distress, however, is also important in the continuing development of the cancer into a larger cancer that will eventually be diagnosed.

Cancer cells are born as a product of abnormal cell division, and they are mostly found in the skin, the mucous membranes, and in the glands. These are the areas of the body where there is the largest turnover of cells; cells that wear out and die, and that have to be replaced.

The skin and mucous membranes of the respiratory, digestive, urinary, and genital tracts are our natural barriers against the environment, while the glands are actively involved in our interaction with it. These natural barriers form our first line of defence against any invasion from outside: against infection. Infection is an invasion of our organism by any foreign material.

Cancer cells appear as an accident of cell division, and this may happen as a spontaneous accident during the critical process of the sharing out of the genetic material, or as a provoked accident by some chemical or virus, or by radioactive particles. The cancer cells then begin to multiply rapidly by doubling.

The word cancer is reserved for the malignant (bad) tumours, the ones that can become a danger to the organism. The other types of tumour are benign ones that rarely cause problems, unless they are located in critical areas, or because of their size.

There is more to say about the cause of cancer. We shall illustrate this by imagining a factory where cars are being produced on an assembly line. Each car that is made in this factory is subjected to strict quality control; defective cars likewise, are destroyed as soon as they are produced.

Once a cancer cell has been born, it should be subject to the vital controls that protect us from infections.

That is what happens normally. Quality checking is performed by a network of controls in the organism which is responsible for making sure that everything proceeds as it should, in order to maintain life. This extensive network is called a *regulating system.* It is an internal servicing system that looks after quality control in the body, defends against invaders, and heals (repair and maintenance).

When cancer cells are born, something must have gone wrong with the normal genetic material of the cells. This abnormal interference could either have come from inside the genes or from outside. Questions usually asked are: was it a hereditary or even accidental defect in the genetic code that was passed on, or was it some outside influence such as chemical pollution that produced the defects by changing the genetic information? Could a virus have entered the cell, and be playing tricks with its genetic material? These questions concern the birth of the cancer cell, its first appearance in normal tissue.

We must also ask, however, what could have happened to the strict quality control at the time of cell division. Why was this regulation system not performing properly to protect the normal cells as it usually does? Was this controlling unit itself somehow compromised? Did some kind of interference make it so carelessly and dangerously inefficient? These questions deal with the quality of infection control.

The state of this regulating system is the other aspect of the coin of what causes cancer. As with any infection (and we shall see that cancer is basically an infection of the body from inside) there are always two sides to this old story: the aspect of the invader (bacteria, viruses, parasites, cancer cells) and that of the invaded organism, the host, that must resist it.

This is a tale of battle. An invader tries to enter, but the host resists: it defends itself against the invader with natural barriers (our skin and mucous membranes that cover the host) and weapons (the inflammation and immune responses).

When does the personality become important in such infection control? Only when it is under lasting severe stress, because:

• Certain personalities are more prone to stress than others.

• Stress is an immune-suppressant; it reduces the efficiency of the regulation network by disorganising it.

What stress really means, in practical terms, we shall discuss later.

Let us put all this more directly with two questions, and give a short answer to each:

(a) Can stress cause an accident with the genetic information of normal cells, so that this produces abnormal cells?

ANSWER: This is unlikely, because, as far as we know, it is an accident in a purely routine biological event.

(b) Can stress in vulnerable personalities cause a suppression of the normally very strict quality control of checking and eliminating?

ANSWER: Very likely. Stress disorganises the entire living system and interferes with the proper efficiency of regulation, with infection control and with healing.

It is the second point that we discuss in this book.

There are many questions that show we are still baffled by the complexity of what is happening in these tiny regions of the body. We are in somewhat the same situation as a programmer who wants to fix a bug in the software program, but who does not understand enough, as yet, of the more subtle details of the programming language. The fine details about cancer are still very much a mystery.

We don't know, for example, why certain races have a tendency to develop certain types of cancers, or why immune suppressive drugs appear to create the risk of developing only certain types of cancer. The risk of cancer increases with age, and it takes time for a cell to complete the malignant transformation from a good cell to a cancer cell (neoplastic change), so that time, and probably a rhythmic repetition of exposure, plays an important role (Deelman effect).

The more malignant cancer cells are, the more they resemble brash and uncontrolled embryonic cells. They become primitive cells both in their appearance and behaviour. They are primitive in that such cells have a strong urge to multiply without restraint, and to stray, to invade, without control. These cells behave like delinquents that avoid the normal rules and regulations of conduct of cell societies. It is as if there has been a return, a regression, to a more primitive and still lawless level of existence, so that they seem to have escaped from the controls that keep cells in their adult mode of behaviour, and in their proper place.

It is better to have a clear idea of the general picture than to go into impractical and uncertain detail because we could easily get lost in details now, and lose sight of the overall biological picture.

We should get one thing clear: having cancer is not the kind of problem for which one can blame oneself. We can never be personally responsible for having cancer, because it is the meeting of a variety of factors that are responsible for its birth. Blaming oneself is unnecessary, and entirely useless.

Stress by itself does not cause cancer. Nor can this type C personality by itself lead to the development of cancer. It will require the combination of enduring severe stress and a suitable personality to produce the disorganisation that goes deep enough to impair normal quality control.

The personality itself is a product of an interweaving of a constitution (everything that we bring with us at birth) and the environment. Our constitution is the more important of the two, something that Freud himself never denied. The birth of the cancer cell is a complex affair, and never a personal one, so that it is ridiculous to say 'it is my own fault'.

The wrong combination of personality and situation can promote the further growth of cancer by interfering with the normal regulations of cell division. It seems unlikely though that the combination can cause the genetic information itself to change. The combination of the wrong personality in the wrong situation can only have an effect if the cancer cells are already present. It can then only allow them to grow by continuing to suppress this function of quality control.

The disturbance inside the organism that can be produced by a meeting of this personality and the stress situation may be so serious that it interferes with the normal recovery processes including defence and healing. Cell division and quality control are part and parcel of this internal servicing system.

We know from everyday experience in general practice that stress impairs the defensive and healing processes to varying degrees. People under stress become sick more often, and their illness will be more severe and last much longer. It takes more time for this patient to recover, and this patient usually has a certain vulnerable personality. It is a stress-prone personality, a double prescription patient; one lot of antibiotics, when needed, is rarely enough.

THE THREE STAGES OF CANCER

We may distinguish three stages of cancer growth:

In the first stage we have the situation in which the cancer is born because of some biological accident. The cells have been allowed to stay alive because of a failure of the quality control of normal cell production at their birth.

The second stage determines whether this early cancer will be allowed to grow into a clinically diagnosed cancer. This stage begins with the quality control. It is a story of infection control, and how good this happens to be.

Stress (in a suitable personality) may be an important factor in allowing the cancer to increase itself so much that it produces symptoms. This is the clinical stage of cancer.

Stress, combined with this cancer-prone personality, can also have a further influence on what happens to the cancer when it is diagnosed. This negative effect does not stop with the birth and diagnosis of the cancer.

The third stage is the course of cancer after the diagnosis has been established, and it is the stage where we begin our description of the typical cancer patient or TCP.

If we accept that stress can cause deep disturbances, then we must state more clearly what we mean by stress. This kind of stress must be something extreme to be so bad for our health. And precisely what we shall have to do, is to see why it is so bad.

When an abnormal cell is created, it takes some time for it to grow to a state in which it can produce clinical symptoms. This is a latency period, a silent time span in which our own organism still has the opportunity to kill it.

(There is another latency period, which is the time it takes for a normal cell to become overtly malignant – neoplastic change – as the result of interference with genetic information, but that does not concern us here.)

In the silent period called the incubation period in infections, the organism detects the presence of the invader and organises itself for battle. During this time the invader continues to multiply and tries to enter deeper into the organism's territory.

Regulation is a biological term for the housekeeping system in the body. It is the task of this housekeeping system to make sure that everything runs normally. Repair, maintenance, and healing, are only three of its functions, and we may say that this regulating system is the general manager that supervises all living processes in the body, and keeps them on the right track.

Our nervous system is a complicated network involved in such regulation and is extended by a system of chemical messengers. If there is an infection, an invasion of the body by foreign material, the regulating system tries to get rid of it. It is usually successful and we take that for granted. During serious stress, however, the regulating system may not be in good working order. Things may go wrong and the system may fail. The invasion of our organism may succeed, so that we develop clinical symptoms of this abnormal situation.

Symptoms of an invasion can vary according to the kind of foreign invader material that is involved. Invaders such as bacteria raise a strong alarm response on invasion, while viruses don't advertise their presence so boldly, preferring to sneak into the cells.

With any breakdown of the normal regulation of the body, the failure to resist and to control an invasion will always have two roots: a body root, and a root in the emotional mind. This means that it is not only the body that fails in its defensive capacity, but that the emotional mind plays its important part in the drama as well. Emotional stress reduces our overall resistance to illness, including our general resistance to cancer. This fact is now almost universally recognised and accepted.

Such enduring stress may continue to do its harmful work after the diagnosis has been made. You may, in the earlier stages of cancer, be more at risk of dying from wrong beliefs than from the cancer.

THE DIAGNOSIS HAS BEEN MADE

We are now going to follow what typically happens after cancer is suspected by the local doctor and the specialist. Let us invent a person, say Mr TCP (as described earlier), and follow him as he goes back to see the specialist for the results of the tests that were done. Mr TCP has spent long days or weeks waiting with apprehension, fearing the results will show that he does have cancer. It is with some fear and trembling that he now waits for the specialist to see him. But he tries to hide it because he is generally not a person who is very open about his feelings. He looks calm enough on the outside, while his wife, who came with him for support, anxiously fiddles with her wedding ring while they wait.

To the patient's fearful emotional mind the ordinary specialist is now no longer an ordinary human doctor, but is a higher judge who will soon decide whether he is going to live or die.

This is how his emotional mind experiences it, even if his rational mind knows that this is not so. And if the emotional mind that feels is at odds with the rational mind that knows, it will always be the emotional mind that wins out because it is more primitive and powerful. The rational mind only offers advice and criticism and remains silent when emotions run high.

As he sits there hoping that the specialist will not give him bad news, Mr TCP is in the grip of intense anxiety. This intense feeling is a hypnosis-like state of the emotional mind in which he is highly suggestible. His rational mind has now taken the back seat. His emotional mind is in such a state that it is ready to believe anything, accept any suggestion, and swallow it without hesitation.

The specialist comes out to him with a serious face, and poor Mr TCP, who is watching the doctor's face anxiously, already knows: 'That's it then.' The surgeon utters those fateful words: 'I'm sorry to tell you, Mr TCP, that you have cancer.' Mr TCP feels a deep sense of despair in his emotional mind, because 'everyone knows that if you've got cancer, that's it, you're finished, that's the end isn't it, you've had it.'

Does Mr TCP say all this out loud, or become hysterical? Not likely. He tries to smile, and asks quietly: 'What are my chances?' or even worse: 'How long do you think I have, doctor?' If he does not ask such questions, he thinks them.

And what does it mean, that he has asked such questions? It means that his emotional mind has accepted a death sentence. His rational mind may tell him a different story but that kind of reasoning does not count in the world of strong feelings. When we worry we tell ourselves that it is no good worrying. Yet that does not stop it.

The specialist may not be aware enough that all this is taking place. He is more concerned with the body than the mind of his patient. This specialist may think he or she is being honest and realistic and that being blunt is required by law. You must not hide anything from the patient.

The sympathetic surgeon is not emotionally involved, except for his pity for Mr TCP and he talks to his patient on a rational level. He is talking about a biological cancer, while a psychological cancer is now invading Mr TCP's emotional mind. It is more dangerous than the biological cancer at this stage.

In his high anxiety, Mr TCP was already in a hypnosis-like state of mind as he sat down to wait, and this state of mind is highly vulnerable to invasion. He will now take suggestions for certainty.

He asks, if he asks at all, the typical first question: 'How long have I got?' He is a good boy, and does not ask too many questions, because he does not want to be difficult.

The surgeon answers: 'You have about six months, Mr TCP, perhaps longer if we can find suitable treatment for you.'

The sentence has been passed: 'six months' is now lodged in his head like a hypnotic instruction, and guess what? He may die in six months unless he manages to break the hypnotic spell. And then he will be in the statistics as having died from cancer, although he may actually have died from a self-produced voodoo death. Mr TCP will in all probability have died from a malignant psychological cancer.

Fortunately, not everyone is like Mr TCP, who will now, after his sentencing, prepare himself emotionally to die at the appointed time, bravely, without making a fuss. Making a fuss is not his style. What has happened now to Mr TCP? He has unwittingly allowed himself to be bone-pointed. After the diagnostic interview, he is being bone-pointed from three different directions. No wonder he has little chance of surviving unless he realises what is happening to him, and does something about it.

First, there is the surgeon who, unknowingly, gave him a death sentence, and who may unwittingly continue, by a thoughtless word or casual gesture, to give him the death sign at every visit. So much so, that most cancer patients become afraid of seeing the specialist again, afraid of what he'll say. If he is referred to a medical or radiological oncologist, this may also continue without anybody being aware of it. The over-sensitivity of Mr TCP to anything that may remind him of what he has accepted as his fate, is hard to imagine for anyone without psychiatric experience. Under the influence of very intense emotions we regress to a more primitive state of consciousness, in which we become aware of the world around us as a world in which people 'give the signs' that confirm our worst fears. This altered state is not so far removed from a delusional state. We are all familiar with lesser effects of such heightened sensitivity: a little girl has a new dress, and feels that the whole world is looking at her, while she preens and prances as she walks. When we are very tense, we may get an uncomfortable feeling that a sudden laugh somewhere is aimed at us, and we make a discrete check if everything is straight and buttoned, even though our rational mind tells us not to be silly. A sensitised person will find references to his or her problems just about everywhere.

Second, Mr TCP, the typical cancer patient, keeps bone-pointing himself, by feeling certain that he must die, and by becoming preoccupied with this notion that he must die, that staying alive is no longer possible. He continually reminds himself of his fate and keeps up the hypnotic instruction.

Third, the bone-pointing comes from everyone else around, from the immediate family to friends and relatives. Friends who have not been around for years now come to visit to remind Mr TCP of his fate, because they have tears in their eyes when they hold his hands in sympathy, don't they? Aren't they really saying (this is how the emotional mind sees it) goodbye?

The impact of our social environment on our emotional well-being can be considerable. If one person tells us we are stupid, we may ignore it. If a second person repeats it, we become somewhat concerned. When a third person mentions it, we begin to question ourselves. We begin to believe it, because we have become sensitised to the idea.

Mr TCP is now in a critical situation. Everything and everyone around him serves to remind him of what is in store. He develops the conviction in his emotional mind that there is no hope at all for him, he might as well face it, he is slated to die. And without hope he cannot survive, because hope is the antidote, the proper medicine, for this wrong setting of his emotional mind. If he does not wake up from this hypnotic state, he will die and prove the statistics right. How true are statistics anyway, when such vulnerable people have been told when to die?

We must make a distinction between a bone-pointed (voodoo or psychogenic) death, and death due to other more mechanical medical complications of cancer.

Biological cancer is an infection, an unauthorised invasion of the body. This, like all other infections, is usually overcome without complications, because we have powerful defensive mechanisms. The immune surveillance system, which is geared to detecting invasions of the body, will detect the presence of these alien cancer cells and get rid of them. Sometimes there arises a complication (which can happen with any other kind of infection); this is when it grows into a clinical cancer. The complication, as with complications in other illnesses, is usually promoted, if not actually provoked, by stress.

The word cancer, in the mind of the lay public, conjures up the image of a powerful monster that will kill you once it has grabbed hold of you. It is the word that is the killer, this wrong belief about cancer, that is so dangerous when left to grow uncontrolled in the emotional mind. That word cancer is the real cancer.

What cancer represents biologically we discuss later. In short, it is an infection that can lead to complications.

The notion of a cancer of the mind is nothing new: Dr Karl Menninger, in his book *The Vital Balance*, writes (page 44) that such a wrong word brings a new kind of fear; not a fear of the actual disease, but of what is incorrectly implied about it in this word. The word cancer, Menninger continues, is said to kill some patients who would otherwise not have died so quickly from it.

What I am saying is this: you don't have to die from cancer, and people may die unnecessarily and prematurely from this wrong word, which is a wrong belief that produces a wrong mental set. This death becomes almost a certainty, because Mr TCP keeps actively working on it until it takes effect. And he does not even know this, because it takes place in his emotional mind.

In effect, Mr TCP now continues the hypnotic instruction (that he allowed himself to receive at the time of diagnosis) by an ongoing process of self-hypnosis. He will therefore maintain his fatal hypnosis to the end.

Our emotional mind is a mind for doing, as Henri Bergson pointed out, for action and not for knowing. It pushes us into what we have to do, it does not make it known to us simply because this is not biologically necessary. When a parent tells a young child to do something, the child simply obeys. It is only later, when the child has already developed a knowing consciousness, a knowing mind, that it will first ask: 'Why?'

Mr TCP must therefore be made aware of this wrong emotional set that may otherwise silently lead him to death, so that he may take counter-measures.

Death from the biological cancer is anything but certain, especially when it is not being assisted and promoted by the patient. When cancer cells arise, they are killed off, just as bacteria are eliminated; when clinical cancer comes as a complication, even then it is not at all certain that anyone has to die from such a complication.

The same emotional factors that are already present before a final diagnosis has been made, may now put the patient in the right frame of mind for the hypnotic instruction: to soften him up as it were, to prepare him for the death sentence and for a totally unnecessary voodoo death.

The emotional factors that come as extras, after the diagnosis has been given, begin their work of making him die a psychosomatic death. Psychogenic death is not rare, it is only rarely recognised. In the next chapter we shall see what can happen to Mr TCP in the days that follow the diagnosis of that complication of the cancer infection that we call clinical cancer.

Chapter Three

THE DEMORALISED PATIENT
GOES HOME

Having come home, and having gone through the expressions of commiseration from those in his social environment, Mr TCP, the typical cancer patient, now allows himself to experience fully that the situation is hopeless. He feels powerless. There is nothing that he himself can do about his cancer; he can't get at it himself, and has to helplessly suffer its presence inside his body. He has to rely on the medical profession for treatment. Nobody can help him, least of all himself.

The initial shock may give him a sense of unreality: 'I can't believe this is happening to me, why me.' When this numbing shock begins to wear off, he finds his problem intolerable, and he feels angry and restless and that he needs to escape from it. But there is no way out; there is nowhere to escape to. He simply can't do anything about it. Whether he knows it or not, he feels trapped, and becomes afraid of his own mind that keeps coming back to this bad news. He rebels against the fact of having cancer. Why me, of all people?

When, later, he resigns himself to his terrible fate, he will become a passive patient who feels useless: he feels helpless and hopeless. He becomes a patient, he feels totally dependent on the medical profession. He thinks that his life is totally in their hands. Mr TCP does not know the difference between treatment and healing.

Mr TCP is now in a highly sensitised and vulnerable state of mind, in which he needs hope more urgently than he needs to be confronted with the idea of dying. He cannot resign himself rationally to such a fate. If he does become resigned to it, the resignation is born out of sheer apathy. It is therefore very important that neither Mr TCP nor those around him feel he must hurriedly come to terms with dying and death. This would contribute strongly to the bone-pointing problem that he is already exposed to.

This confrontation with the spectre of dying is inappropriate in this situation, because he is not in a proper frame of mind for being rational. It is the wrong time for it. He is in deep despair, he is depressed, and may later even become apathetic: emotionally numb, without any interest in anything, a psychological vegetable. How can he be open to sober reason?

Mr TCP is now in a state of complete demoralisation; a state of mind that consists of feelings of helplessness, hopelessness, and despair. He has been softened up for defeat, and he is ready for an untimely death, a psychogenic death.

Dr Menninger, an eminent American psychiatrist, described the state of mind of chronic psychotic patients (a psychosis is a seriously disorganised state of the emotional mind) and then commented: what could be worse than this? Can any personality get worse than that? The answer, wrote Menninger, is simply yes.

This worse state of mind is the pitiful clinical picture of a psychogenic death. This is a death that has been motivated by suggestions, based on wrong beliefs. (*The Vital Balance*, pages 262, 263).

This is precisely the state of mind of the demoralised cancer patient, and unless he is helped out of it, he is doomed.

Psychogenic means brought about by the mind. We don't say caused by the mind, because a cause belongs to physics; this physical cause is not the same as an emotional cause, which is a motive, and is based on emotional logic. What may be impossible from a rational point of view, may be feasible according to emotional logic.

Emotional logic goes where rational logic turns back. We can think in rational logic, but our body runs on emotional logic, which is the logic of life itself. Our reasoning mind could be sceptical about the possibility of dying from an intensely wrong belief, but our emotional mind can find nothing impossible in that.

Psychogenic death is also known as psychosomatic death, and as taboo or voodoo death. The method of dying may be spontaneous, which is to say that we don't know how it is done, or, more usually, brought about with assistance.

How such people die, cannot be explained by physical causes and by rational logic. It happens through emotional logic, the logic that holds the power over life and death, through an emotional instruction that organises the person for death.

This assistance in a psychogenic death is an important point for consideration, because such assistance can be:

(a) Self-assistance: Mr TCP keeps reminding himself that he is finished. He visualises himself into a psychogenic death; to death by self-instruction. If we feel that this is an exaggerated statement, we need only remind ourselves of the feats of self-hypnotic visualisation that have been recorded. This self-induced hypnotic state is present in conditions of religious fervour, in which we see many examples of bleeding from symbolically significant locations, such as the Christian stigmata of bleeding from the palms and feet, and around the forehead (crown of thorns). This fervour represents an absolute belief, a conviction, an identification, becoming one, with the figure of Christ or other deity.

It is this absolute certainty in religious ecstasy and other forms of emotional hypnosis that makes it possible. Kroger, in his book on clinical and experimental hypnosis, states (page 136) that if a suggestion becomes a conviction, it has the power to produce an appropriate response in the body. He goes on to say: 'It is known that, in the presence of an appropriate mental set, thoughts based on conviction can heal or kill.' We add that these thoughts are emotional issues and not rational-theoretical considerations.

(b) Assistance by social environment: This includes family and relatives, friends, doctors, nursing staff, and others. The people around him say or think or act out: 'You poor thing', and Mr TCP is well aware that they check him to see if he is already looking terrible. Everybody around reminds him that he has cancer, and that having cancer means he is finished.

Even if they don't know it, their ongoing suggestion to him, when he is already so highly vulnerable to negative thinking and visualising, has a powerful emotional effect. It hammers in the bad message and keeps working.

All this works through emotional logic. The condition of mind that leads to this totally unnecessary psychogenic death is that of complete demoralisation, and this is a serious illness that usually goes unrecognised. If Mr TCP dies, this cause of his death goes unrecognised, and his death will be assigned to the cancer.

This dangerous sickness of the emotional mind leads the person to passively await death. Such a death is not the result of a wilful, deliberate, self-killing, but of a demoralised get-it-over-and-done-with attitude of total despair. It is the 'give-up-itis' that has been recorded in prisoners of war and civilians in concentration camps, who have given up all hope of surviving. Mr TCP then abandons himself completely to the conviction of dying, which activates the proper programme for dying.

The state of mind that is necessary for a psychosomatic death, and the social conditions that promote it, are not rare, only not sufficiently recognised. It is important to identify such sick persons, because this death can be prevented; it is an unnecessary death.

The thoroughly demoralised cancer patient suffers from this abnormal mental set, that is based on the wrong conviction that she or he must die from cancer, that death is inevitable. In their minds there is no alternative to dying; surviving is no longer an option.

Such patients allow themselves to be bone-pointed by their social environment. They have accepted a terribly wrong belief system that has been pushed on to them by others. They are convinced it is true. They lose hope, feel helpless, sink into deep despair, and die unnecessarily. It is not the cancer that kills them, but the voodoo curse that has, unwittingly, been placed on them.

This premature psychogenic death is a self-generated and socially assisted death. Who are the able assistants? Lay public opinion, doctors, nursing staff, family, and friends, acquaintances, and casual contacts.

Jerome Frank, a professor of psychiatry, wrote an important book on persuasion and healing, and he quotes (page 52) from a paper by Warner: 'A victim's expectation of death may be powerfully reinforced by the attitudes of his group'. How powerful? Dr Frank quotes from the same paper a description of the way a man of a North Australian Aboriginal tribe died through a tribe-assisted tradition. When a person's soul has been stolen and the theft becomes known, he and his tribe collaborate in speeding him to his death. If he has lost his soul, he is already half dead, and his family and friends treat him as already dead, so that he obligingly dies soon after. The man is convinced he must die, that the situation is hopeless and he is in deep despair. This wrong belief system is supported by his tribe, by those around him who are close to him. This has a strong effect on him.

Such powerful strategies of punishment may differ in content in different social environments, but the effect is the same. How powerful this social impact can be on the emotional mind of any person is illustrated by the following report from Colin Turnbull, an experienced field anthropologist, who once offended a village witch doctor in the Congo.

Turnbull wrote that he was at first amused by the witchcraft that was used against him by the village witch doctor. As a veteran researcher, he was not prone to primitive superstition. The entire village now treated him as if he did not exist; they ignored him or only spoke to each other in his presence about the curse that had been placed on him by the local witch doctor. In this way they kept reminding him that his fate was sealed.

In spite of himself, he began to feel sick. He started to vomit, and felt extremely weak. At the same time he (his rational mind) was aghast at the absurd fact that he, an Oxford graduate, was becoming the victim of an African native curse. His rational-logical mind was unable to save him, and he could only survive by producing counter magic on the advice of some sympathetic pygmies. (A. Neher, *The psychology of transcendence*, pages 1 and 2).

Rational logic says it can't be true, but emotional logic is what makes it happen, and the rational mind eventually becomes silent, and retreats to a back seat.

How does all this relate to doctors? Imagine the following scene: Mr TCP and his wife have come to the rooms for the results of the tests, and the surgeon calls them in. The surgeon, solemnly: 'I'm sorry to tell you, Mr TCP, that you've got a malignancy there, and I fear that it is too late for an operation.'

Mr TCP feels his courage ebbing away, but he says bravely: 'Oh, well, you can't win them all, I s'pose doctor. How long have I got?' Surgeon: 'Well, I can't give you more than three months, Mr TCP. I'm sorry to say it, but I don't think that you will see Christmas.' On a rational level of communication this is objective information, but in the way Mr TCP hears it, it is pure bone-pointing: a hypnotic instruction to die at the indicated time.

As soon as he and his tearful wife are out of the door, his wife breaks out crying, and falls into his arms: 'Oh, John, I'm so sorry. Poor John, whatever are we going to do?' The social bone-pointing by family and friends begins.

Coming home with the bad news, everybody cries and hugs

him, and soon family and relatives, his friends, and even long forgotten friends who have heard the bad news, come to visit, all with long faces, hugging him or shaking his hands, with tears in their eyes. In a particularly perceptive moment Mr TCP called this 'a funeral atmosphere'. Indeed it is; they are in effect all saying goodbye to him.

Mr TCP once said angrily of such behaviour: 'Everybody keeps reminding me that I am dying, and I feel every bloody handshake is a nudge in the wrong direction. They're like a bunch of grave diggers.' What he is saying here is this: nobody treats him like an ordinary citizen any more, and he is now a marked man who gets 'special treatment' from his social tribe. He is a man marked for death.

And what of the oncologist whom Mr TCP is seeing soon after? 'He shakes his head a bit every time he sees my card, and he pulls a grave face, you get it doc? Every time I think I feel much better, he says: I don't want to raise any false hopes, Mr TCP, it doesn't look too good, you know.'

Mr TCP falls mentally into a heap, and is back into despair, and begins to experience a growing phobia about the oncologist, and for any other doctor who might bring him more bad news. He feels like avoiding them now, because he has become over-sensitive, allergic, to bad news.

Wherever he goes socially, the moment he comes in, there is a sudden short silence, and then everyone becomes artificially cheerful. Pretty soon Mr TCP begins to look awful, he loses weight, his skin colour becomes pale, grey and yellowish, and there is no question that he looks terminal. Poor Mr TCP. What chance has he got, unless someone rescues him from this untimely psychogenic death? Is this so different from the example of the psychogenic death of the North Australian tribesman? Isn't Mr TCP's dilemma also a process of socially assisted dying?

And how did Mr TCP fare? His first words to me were: 'I've got terminal cancer doc,' and breaks out crying.

'He cries all the time, doctor,' says his wife, 'poor man, I don't know what to do with him. He doesn't eat, he's lost all interest, just doesn't want to do anything any more.'

'Who says you're terminal?'

'What, doc?'

'Who says you are terminal?'

'The oncologist, he said that to me when he saw me, he thinks I am a hopeless case, I know, I'm finished.' (This was his own interpretation, not the voiced opinion of the oncologist.)

'Look here, Mr TCP, he can't possibly tell you that you are terminal unless he claims he's got extrasensory perception, and can see the future, and he would never claim that. What he means is that, always and only statistically speaking, an average case like yours has such and such a survival limit. He is not talking about you at all, he is only talking about Mr Average, about statistics.'

How reliable are these statistics? How many people recover and don't go back to enter the statistics, and how many people die obligingly to fit them?

A surgeon told a patient that she should not think of going on her long holiday overseas, and this wonderful lady retorted: 'Doctor, you may know your statistics, but you don't know *me.*' With such an attitude, is it a wonder that she survived?

I explain to Mr TCP the difference between a statistical average and a unique single case. A statistical average can never be a certainty for the unique individual. What may seem hopeless according to a statistical average, is never a cinch in the unique case, in which there is always hope.

Mr TCP began to understand, and did well because he threw off the dying spell of the psychological cancer. It was a load off his mind. He began to realise that he now had hope, which is to say that he had, at least, a fighting chance in the battle with the biological cancer. His death was not certain, and he had a chance to survive. This is an entirely different picture from his previous state, in which the fight was not even an option. Then, he was already beaten because he could not even start a fight.

Mr TCP became cheerful again, he put on weight, and began to look healthy again. He started to take an interest in his environment again, to the surprise of his oncologist, who merely shook his head again and cautiously advised: it's only a temporary remission, don't hope for too much. But Mr TCP was now no longer sensitive to this.

The doctor is not wilfully negative, we must understand, he must cover himself, because he is under a legal obligation to tell the unvarnished truth. Unfortunately, his idea of the honest truth may be an uneducated one, not taking into account that the future is never certain.

A truth without any hope is therefore never the real truth, but merely a harsh sentence.

Doctors and relatives may badly misjudge a patient's capacity to carry the crushing knowledge of having cancer because, as the French satirist La Rochefoucauld scoffed: we can all find the strength to bear up under someone else's misfortune.

Added to this is the doctor's reliance on medical technique, so that he may have lost sight of the natural capacity of the organism to defend itself, and of the impact that an emotional mind can have on this natural capacity for healing. He may therefore ignore the patient's own capacity for defence and healing to support his efforts.

There are better oncologists, of course, who are more informed and therefore sympathetic and supportive, and hold out hope, and encourage their patients to become actively involved in the fight and to make this fight their own fight.

Some conservative doctors suffer from an outdated medical philosophy that denies the patient's emotional mind can have any useful input in her or his own illness (more about this in the introductory chapter and chapter thirty-one).

Menninger (same book) describes the history of a woman with a chronic psychosis, who suddenly recovered because a doctor became interested in her case, and did his best to help her. For many years she had vegetated in an institution as a hopeless chronic case. This is what happens so often with such chronic patients, wrote Menninger; the patient, and her relatives, and, worst of all, the physicians, accepted her case in passive resignation as being hopeless. Her pitiful state of mind, itself the result of this wrong attitude of people around her, is known as institutionalisation. However, we don't have a proper word for the harmful state of mind which is present in the family and the doctors.

This state of mind, Menninger went on, 'is of the utmost malignancy', because it assumes the situation is totally hopeless. Everyone gives up hope: 'No one has any expectation that anything will make any difference. Death is patiently, helplessly, hopelessly awaited' (page 347). The social attitude may be unwitting, but fatally effective for all that.

If there is no chemotherapy available, and radiotherapy or

surgery is not indicated, a sympathetic oncologist may think that a patient feels reassured by saying: 'Mr TCP, I won't let you suffer.' From an objective no-nonsense point of view, this is a kind and reassuring statement to make. But Mr TCP says he felt a cold shiver on hearing these words, without knowing why. What is the significance of this cold shiver? It tells us that his over-sensitive emotional mind has responded to the emotional meaning in this reassurance. His rational mind did not even know what was going on. In terms of emotional logic it is as if the oncologist had said: 'Because there is no physical treatment for you, you have no hope of surviving; but don't worry, I will ease you out'.

Professor Frank (same book, page 47) pointed out that the insensitivity of scientific medicine to the bad effects of wrong emotions is probably responsible for many failures, and it motivates patients to look elsewhere for forms of treatment which are based on a healthier attitude. These alternative helpers focus on mobilising or strengthening the patient's natural healing powers.

And what is this healing power on which these alternative helpers dare to bet? It is the *vis medicatrix naturae*, the spontaneous healing force of nature. We rarely hear this expression in modern medicine, wrote Menninger (page 366), even when we rely on it every day; how would a wound ever heal without it? Yet, many medical experts take the sole credit for this natural push for spontaneous healing.

Without this natural healing force no life is possible because it is the moving force of life itself. We heal without being asked. We heal by default, if we will let mother nature do her work properly and, particularly, if we actively support her in her efforts, and don't hamper her by having a wrong mindset.

At the time of diagnosis, the patient is in a hypnosis-like (hypnoid) state, brought about by the intense anxiety. In this unstable emotional state of high suggestibility, the sentence 'You have cancer' is heard as a death sentence: 'You must die.' This is no exaggeration; the behaviour of many patients expresses this quite clearly.

Mr TCP's acceptance of the death sentence as a hypnotic instruction is confirmed by the question that is so often the first one, and it does not matter whether it is spoken or only thought: 'How long have I got?'

What kind of question is this? The doctor, being emotionally uninvolved, may only hear a rational inquiry about time, and advises the patient to enjoy every day, little realising how cruel this is. The patient is really saying: 'I have accepted my sentence, and I just want to know when I must go'. To say 'Enjoy every day' is saying: hurry, because the time is all too near. Unschooled sympathy can hurt.

Unless the patient is rescued from his hypnotic instruction to die, the obliging patient will proceed to die an untimely psychosomatic death at approximately the appointed time. This is the patient who makes little fuss on the outside, who can't make a fuss, and dies quietly, without audible protest. This poor patient exists in essentially the same situation as the tribesman who has been bone-pointed, and who is now hastened to his death by his social environment.

Let me repeat that not all cancer patients ask this fateful question, only the TCPs. One patient even joked: 'My wife wants to know what is the risk that I might survive, doctor.'

Chapter Four

BATTLE FATIGUE

We have seen how Mr TCP becomes demoralised soon after the diagnosis of his cancer. Let us now look at a second form of demoralisation which can occur much later, and in a different personality. This emotional disorder may appear in a person who rallies from the initial shock of the diagnosis, and is more or less determined to fight for recovery. The more determined this patient is to take an active hand in the process of recovery, the less likely is it that battle fatigue will occur, but even the best soldier may get sick and tired of fighting on.

Here are some of the emotional pressures that the patient has to endure. It is easy to see that they can accumulate to become an emotional overload.

When the patient feels herself (or himself) to be only a helpless and passive bystander in the struggle between oncologist and cancer, without being actively involved in the fight, then the emotional problem may occur earlier than in the determined fighter.

Daily confrontation with uncertainty is a major factor in the appearance of the battle fatigue syndrome.

The drawn-out struggle with the cancer eventually leaves the patient emotionally exhausted, worn-out and weary from trying to cope, for so long, with both the biological and psychological cancers.

This struggle also involves the following:

(a) The scary idea of having cancer, and the threatening and discouraging uncertainty of recovery.

(b) Weakening and sickening side effects of repeated bouts of chemotherapy or radiotherapy, or repeated surgery.

(c) Fear of tests and their results.

(d) Surrounding funereal social atmosphere at the start of the diagnosis makes way for an ill-concealed impatience with the chronic sufferer.

Even members of the close family lose patience after a while with the person who is sick all the time, and who needs so much attention. Long-term illness is rarely well tolerated, although at the start, the support coming from the same persons may be wonderful.

The patient begins to feel a burden on the family; the illness may become a financial burden; the illness disrupts the normal routine of living. When the initial crisis settles somewhat, life only rarely goes back to normal. No matter how much they love the patient, other members of the family often can't help showing irritation and impatience. The poor patient is reminded over and over again of his or her 'nuisance value' by staying alive.

Long weeks and months of chemotherapy or radiotherapy, with their weakening and sickening effects on the body and the emotions of the patient, dread of having to undergo more tests, and yet another bout of treatment, fear of adverse test results, all these have to be faced repeatedly, with no guarantee of success. It is a nightmarish existence. The indignity of the changed appearance, due to surgery or chemo and radiotherapy, plays havoc with the self-image and self-esteem, and may impair it considerably. This, too, leads to loss of self-confidence.

If all this continues too long and too often, emotional fatigue sets in, a battle weariness that makes the patient feel sick and tired of having to keep up the hard struggle, of fighting what is now perceived as a losing fight. Death, which may not have been a real option before, or merely a distant threat, now becomes a distinct possibility. Worse, it may begin to lose its awfulness, and take on the appearance of the ultimate bringer of relief.

This is an emotional illness that would have been recognised and treated, had this patient been a soldier at the front. But in the front line with cancer, this battle fatigue often goes unnoticed and untreated, almost unseen behind the treatment of the biological cancer in the foreground.

This is not Mr TCP, who experiences his demoralisation at the very beginning of the cancer drama, but a person who does not give up immediately, who does not succumb quickly and readily to the myth of dying. This is the person who is willing to fight, if there is sufficient motivation and encouragement.

As the weeks and months go by, and there is no enduring relief from this constant confrontation with uncertainty and struggle with the disease and its treatment, the patient gradually begins to lose heart.

Professor Jores quoted Dr Armand Vincent as saying that doctors generally only try to prevent death and do not help the patient to live. The surgeon, remarked Jores, will remove an ulcer without taking notice of the personal problems which may exist with it, and that remain unsolved (A. Jores: *Der Mensch und seine Krankheit*, page 146).

The patient, as a highly emotional human creature who must undergo such unrelenting stress, seems to be ignored in the battle with the biological cancer. No wonder then that this patient gradually drifts into a state of demoralisation that will reduce resistance to the disease, diminish the will to live and prolong such a poor quality life.

Expressions now begin to surface, such as: 'What's the point, anyway? I'm getting sick and tired of all this. I've had enough, I can't take this misery much longer, I'd rather die.'

And what begins as a complaint in the stress of the struggle, gradually becomes accepted as a real option. This is a problem that is not limited to the battle fatigue regarding cancer, something like it happens in a marital battlefront. An initial idle threat of: 'Maybe we should break up' becomes an option, and then a reality all too readily, if the discord continues without a solution.

The battle fatigue needs to be treated, not accepted. It is a cry of distress. And the cry of need should be heard clearly and loudly.

I read somewhere of a Zen master who said: 'If ever I should find myself threatened, I shall shout loud and long for help.' Cancer patients, take note of that: if the enlightened Zen master sees no reason to keep quiet about his distress, then why should you? Open your mouth really wide, and shout loud and clear if you need help. Never keep a stiff upper lip. Loosen it and make waves with it.

Part Two

THE BIOLOGY
OF CANCER

Chapter Five

THE NATURE OF CANCER

Cancer is an infection of the body, but it is a special kind of infection. The word infection is usually reserved for an invasion of our body by other living organisms, and these may be viruses, bacteria, fungus cells, or parasites. Transplants (grafted tissue) and cancer complete this list of living foreign invaders.

Invasion means that the entry is not supposed to happen, that it happens by accident and is not to our benefit. Each of these micro-organisms can provoke their own specific kind of defensive response from the body, which means that the body deals with them in different ways. There are variations of the same basic defensive response.

Our organism can live in relatively peaceful coexistence with its natural environment of micro-organisms. This is a balanced give-and-take relation that is like a mutual benefit society. It is called a symbiotic relationship. You help me and I'll help you.

Our bowels, for example, house bacteria that live there peacefully. The bacteria return the favour by producing certain vitamins that we use. Bacteria are also allowed to live on our skin, and they protect it from harmful bacteria in return. Such normal bowel and body-surface bacteria are intolerant of other strains of bacteria.

Other micro-organisms are not so peacefully inclined; not only are they of no use to us, they even want to invade us and take over, if they can. Against such opportunistic and harmful invaders, we have a defensive (protective) system that has two departments that must work together: we have a 'department for inflammation responses', as well as a 'department for immune responses'.

The department for inflammation is much older, and is already found in primitive organisms. The department for immune responses is a special unit that is newer in evolution, and is more specifically orientated against particular invaders.

If our body were a country, we would compare the department of inflammation response to the war department or to military intelligence. It is responsible for these three jobs:

(a) It must detect any invasion;

(b) It must send troops to get rid of these invaders;

(c) After that has been accomplished, it calls on the healing department to send the engineer corps for repairs (healing of damage).

The department for immune affairs is a secret service that has the task of detecting and eliminating specific enemy agents. These two intelligence departments work so closely together, that their duties often overlap. Their function is to keep out invaders: to detect and eliminate anything that does not belong in the body.

Invaders can be grouped into two classes:

(a) Inanimate (not alive) invaders, such as thorns, pieces of wood, glass, metal, and chemical irritants. Army intelligence signals the presence of the invaders, and calls on the army to eliminate these. The secret service may not be needed in this general operation.

Chemicals that enter the bloodstream through the digestive tract or by injection, have to pass through the liver, which is a detoxification centre. The liver tries to turn chemicals into harmless substances, which then pass out of the body via the kidneys.

The presence of invading foreign substances such as thorns is usually easily detected, but glass, steel, and special metal alloys, are more difficult to detect. These are fairly inert (chemically neutral) substances, and do not advertise their presence in the body.

(b) Animate invaders. These are bacteria, fungi, and parasites. These invaders are readily detected by army intelligence, and if this fails, there is always the secret service to fall back on. Parasite infestations will often produce an allergic response; but viruses sneak into our cells, so that the symptoms of their invasion may not be immediately obvious.

Our body always tries to inactivate an invader before it can do harm. It may do it through the army (inflammation) or through the secret service (immune response) or through both.

When the army is called to the invaded area, it arrives via the bloodstream, and immediately throws a net around the invader; it then coats this invader with an appetiser called opsonin, which in turn attracts phagocytes: powerful, hungry hunter cells (white blood cells), that gobble up the invaders. We know when this battle is taking place by local signs of infection: swelling, redness, heat, pain, and the loss of function that results from the inflammation.

If the invader is too large, the army may form a tough capsule around it to fence it off, so that the invader cannot do harm or escape.

Fever, malaise, and an increase in the number of fighting units (white blood cells) in the bloodstream, are the general (systemic) signs of the fighting that is going on; the entire organism has now become mobilised for war.

Where does cancer fit in? To understand this better, we must first look at invasions of our body with neutral metal alloys, and then at an invasion by grafting (transplantation).

1. Experience with early prostheses (artificial body parts), has shown that they often draw attention to themselves, so that they are attacked by the body's elimination teams as soon as its intelligence system recognises their foreign nature. The challenge here is to find alloys (metal combinations) that make the prosthesis inert as far as the body is concerned. The most modern prostheses are made up of metal alloys that make them almost undetectable, in the same way that Stealth fighters escape radar detection. Modern hip and knee prostheses, for example, barely advertise their presence and provoke little body response.

2. Tissue transplants; these cells are also rejected by the body, and the rejection means that their presence has already been detected, their foreign nature recognised, and that they have been attacked. Tissue from strangers is rejected out of hand. Therefore organ transplants require massive doses of immune-suppressants to protect them from attack by the immune system. The immune system must be practically put out of action to save the transplant. The result of such suppression of the immune system is, of course, increased risk of infection and malignancy. These immune-suppressive and immune-modifying drugs are also used in auto-immune disorders. Anti-cancer (cytotoxic) drugs have this immune-suppressant effect as an unwanted side-effect of their action on the cancer cells.

Resistance and immunity are the two ways in which our organism insists on its rejection of any foreign material. Our organism protects itself by simply saying a big no! to them.

The more familiar transplanted tissue is to the host (the person suffering the invasion) the less the host protests against the presence of the invader. A healthy rejection of the transplant is the rule, except in the case of uni-ovular twins.

The surface of our body (the skin and the mucous membranes of the airways, digestive, and urinary tract) is designed to naturally resist invaders. This surface is our first line of defence, and is the most frequent site of infection. Also, with our active gland tissue, it is the most frequent site of cancer.

If this defensive barrier has been penetrated, and the invasion is not stopped by local inflammation, the invader will now have the opportunity to spread deeper inwards via the lymph vessels. The invaders are halted at the local lymph glands, which form a second line of defence against invasion. These glands swell in battle, and most people have had some experience with such swellings in the neck, under the arm, or in the groin.

CANCER AS AN INFECTION

Cancer is made up of cells that have come from our own body. They are invaders from inside our own body. As far as our body is concerned, these cells are traitors and outlaws. They are completely useless to our system, and they must be rejected out of hand.

The more malignant the cancer, the more irregular and unruly its cells will be, so that they will become different from their parent cells, and from each other. Some change so drastically that they may resemble cells from a different organ. They may even do similar work. Something has gone wrong with the codes that assign normal cells their form, location and conduct as civilised and useful members of the cellular community.

Here is another strange biological situation: the more malignant a cancer cell is, the more different it should become from the tissue that gives rise to it; therefore it should be detected more quickly and eliminated from the body. Unfortunately, the more the cancer cell varies from its normal parent cells, the more it will refuse to obey the laws that regulate normal tissue cells.

The cancer cell becomes an outlaw cell and takes no notice of the rules for community living that apply to normal cells. The cancer cell becomes mobile and goes where it is not supposed to. We can be sure, however, that when it strays to other tissues which are not its parent tissue, it will not be made welcome, and that it will meet a hostile reception. It is not so easy for cancer cells to survive in a different organ: cancer cells are usually not hardy enough to withstand an intolerant rejection by their new environment.

As a first measure, the growth of the cancer must be stopped. It must be contained before its elimination can begin. To find the cancer cells, stop their growth, and kill them off, is the urgent task of the body's defence system.

Getting rid of the cancer cells is usually no problem for the body, because it has powerful removal mechanisms. The problem seems to lie more in a detection failure:

(a) Some cancers can hide themselves immunologically and thus escape detection. They mask their foreign presence.

(b) Our intelligence services can be depleted or suppressed by various means:

  (i) Sometimes the cancer tissue itself may somehow manage to suppress the intelligence systems.
 (ii) Chemotherapy, radiotherapy, and the administration of drugs like cortisone can do this.
(iii) Stress is a powerful suppressant of both army and secret service intelligence systems. In addition to this, our normally efficient elimination and healing systems will also suffer and become less effective.

This is why it is not always easy for the body to say no to the cancer in the same definite way that it can say no to bacteria and pieces of wood. If only the body would recognise the alien character of the cancer, and treat it as it does a piece of wood or bacterial cells. It is usually the body's secret service (secret intelligence department) that must deal with such stealthy invaders from within, and the department is quite vulnerable to the negative effect of stress.

We know of another instance in which the invasion comes from inside, but it is a pseudo-invasion. We may imagine that the secret intelligence system has become paranoid and overactive, and starts accusing normal citizen cells of being foreign invaders. It calls on the army to destroy these (apparently) perfectly innocent cells. This is known as an auto-immune disease.

Some cancers are so different that they can call up an inflammatory response, which means that the cancer is being attacked by the more primitive and powerful war department. But not all cancers do this. There have been attempts to stimulate this primitive inflammatory response by injecting bacterial vaccines, such as those against tuberculosis, but there are problems with the method that make it less useful.

The message in this chapter is this: think of cancer as being no different from any other infection. We may say that the only difference is that here the invasion comes from inside the body. We have to do everything in our capacity to assist our internal systems in their work of detecting, eliminating, and healing. This means boosting our physical health and emotional well-being so that we can maximise our resistance.

It is now acknowledged that there is a psychological aspect to the cancer problem, and that we have input into this defensive process via our emotional mind. Cancer is now a topic in the newer books on psychiatry, under the heading of psychosomatic medicine.

Diagnosis of cancer should not be a cause for despair, but it is a time for stopping and taking stock of our life so far.

Chapter Six

BASIC BIOLOGY

To understand better what happens, and should happen, in the fight against cancer, we need a little biological background.

Like all other animals, and even insects, our human organism is made up of two main parts: an 'action system' in the front for interacting with the outside world, and a 'support system' for this action system.

In insects such as ants and bees (see figure below), we can see this arrangement quite clearly: in the front there is an action system that has one leading head with sensory organs, and a number of pairs of limbs on the sides. This may be compared to a truck that has the cabin in front, and a trailer attached to it. The trailer is the insect's oval belly in this case. It is like a kitchen which supports the action system and supplies it with food and fuel.

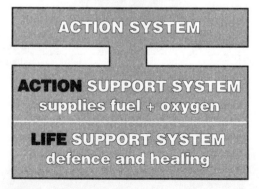

THE WORLD
interaction

ACTION SYSTEM

ACTION SUPPORT SYSTEM
supplies fuel + oxygen

LIFE SUPPORT SYSTEM
defence and healing

The action system interacts with its environment. It is our front line with the world. It has sensory organs to search out the surrounding world for whatever the organism needs and an operating system of limbs to gather all that into itself.

Our front-line system interacts with the world around us. It consists of:

• One leading head equipped with sense organs to give us the necessary information about the environment we have to act on. This sensory equipment is a rather primitive guiding mind; it must decide on what action to take on the basis of that incoming information.

• One or more pairs of limbs (insects and animals may also have wings) to operate on the world. These are conveniently placed behind the leading head: information is followed by action.

In animals, the head leads, so that it is sensibly placed in front of the body, from where it searches out the surrounding world for relevant practical information. In the upright human being the head is placed on top of the operating and support systems, and this is even more efficient, because it surveys the environment from a greater height, so it has a wider vision.

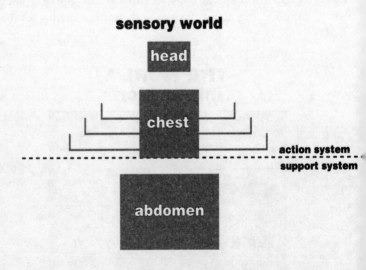

The support system is simply a kitchen for the action system, and located behind it. In higher organisms this is located in the trunk: everything that is between the shoulders and the hips.

In mobile systems, it consists of a fuel uptake system (a digestive system), an oxygen uptake system (a respiratory system), and a circulation system to bring fuel and oxygen to the action system at the front line, and to carry garbage back to the kidneys. And then we have the kidneys as a garbage disposal system. Finally, we have a life-support system for healing and defence as a combined engineering and medical system.

The support system simply supports the actions at the front line, which is the battlefront with the world. It is located behind the action system.

This world is an environment that feeds and shelters us, but it is one from which we must also protect ourselves. It may become inhospitable (too hot, too cold, too dry, too wet etc.) or hostile, threatening to invade us. This environment is our natural habitat, and we have been naturally outfitted with all that we need for coping with it.

To live in the world, we have the following proper equipment:

Sense organs to search for food and shelter, as well as an operating system that allows us to move around in this world, and to take from it what we need.

An internal action-support system that processes food and oxygen for fuel (digestive and respiratory system), and puts back into that world all that we no longer need (excretion system). There is also a circulation system to bring food and fuel around, and to deliver the kitchen garbage to the kidneys for excretion.

A life-support system that has two main departments:

• A department for self-protection: this works to protect and defend us from that world, whenever it becomes inhospitable or hostile. This is our defence system.

• A repair and maintenance department to heal any damage that we may suffer in this process of self-protection. This is our healing system.

To guide the active organism with greater efficiency, many systems have a guiding mind that controls their behaviour by means of sensations (instincts) and emotions; through feelings that work quickly and anonymously. This guiding mind in humans (which we may call our emotional mind), sits in the driver's seat of our organismic wagon, behind the wheel and other controls. It is the practical driver that steers it in the direction of survival.

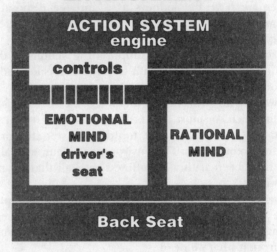

Human beings also have a rational mind: an intellectual mind that is busy with theoretical speculation. This rational mind sits in the passenger's seat, and can only comment and advise the emotional mind on what can be done about things according to rational-theoretical logic.

The emotional mind, however, uses a different logic: an emotional logic. This is the proper logic for both action and practical thinking, which is thinking for immediate action and for the sake of survival. It will ignore the rational mind if it finds that rational-theoretical logic goes against its own emotional logic. This is useful whenever we meet a snake in the bush: we jump away, without stopping to think rationally about the situation. We cannot afford to wait to find out if the snake is poisonous: fear makes us jump before our rational mind knows what is going on. Emotional logic is the effective logic of practical survival.

How do the two forms of mind logic work together?

When we are involved in action, busily doing something, we are that practical emotional mind: we shift into the driver's seat when we have to become bodily active. When some problem comes up during our action then, as we say, we stop to think. This means that we stop being the emotional mind, and we shift into the passenger's seat, while we stop doing whatever we were doing. We now become the rational mind for as long as we need to think things over. When we have solved the problem, and are ready to go on, we become the emotional mind again. These two minds are two different attitudes that we can adopt, like two roles that we can play, but always with only one at a time.

The emotional mind has often acted long before the rational mind could even begin to think. In emergency situations, there is no time to think things over rationally. The quick emotional mind takes charge. It is in charge if there is any doubt who should be boss. If our emotions are too strong, they will prevent the shift to the rational mind.

This dominance is not so useful, and it can even be harmful, if the emotional mind entertains wrong ideas, and sends on wrong instructions. The rational mind advises us to stop smoking, for example. It may recite many rational arguments, reasons, why the organism should stop smoking. But if the emotional mind, for whatever motive, ignores this sound advice, and urges us to go on smoking, the organism will continue to light up. The rational mind then states: 'I know this is wrong, but I can't help it'. It is always helpless against the determined emotional mind in the driver's seat.

When feelings become intense, our rational mind moves to a back seat, from where it can no longer be heard: its advising voice has become faint and powerless, even silent.

All living beings have the capacity to protect themselves from the environment, because this environment may become a hazard to their continuing well-being. It may become inhospitable (in cold or heat) or hostile, threatening to invade the organism. In either case, it threatens to damage the living being.

To protect ourselves from such environmental damage, we have a powerful regulating system that shelters and safeguards our body from harm. This same system also protects us from any accidental internal damage by minimising the disturbance and compensating for any loss of function.

This is a housekeeping or managing system that is run by that complex biological computer that we call our nervous system. This computer is continuously active in keeping our organism going, and staying on track. Our nervous system has the vital task of adapting our organism to the changing environment. It is a highly complex regulating network that stretches beyond the reach of the nerves. Where the nerves end, it makes clever use of chemical messengers to get to the more remote areas.

Our regulating system adapts our organism to any changes that take place in the outside world. This is its first and main task: to support our interaction with our world. This regulating system is first and foremost geared to action. This can be seen from the natural arrangement of our basic nervous system. It has three parts: (i) a sensory part for searching out the world. This consists of our sense organs; (ii) a motor part for operating on that world: this is our bone-supported muscle system; (iii) an action-coordinating and action-supporting part: this is the so called autonomic (self-regulating) nervous system. It may be compared to an administration system that keeps tabs on what goes on, and coordinates activities.

The autonomic nervous system is an internal regulating system that services those organs which support our interaction with the outside world. It also has special units, such as the defence and healing units. Our autonomic system makes use of glands which produce chemical messengers to reach beyond the nerve endings.

THE WORLD

ACTION SYSTEM

REGULATION SYSTEM
- Action support
- Life support and maintenance

These outer and inner regulating systems form one complex unit that continuously monitors and balances our entire organism in its task to survive. We shall simply call this total unit the regulating system. It is easy to see that this forms a vital part of the internal housekeeping that keeps us going.

Our regulating system has (roughly) the following tasks:

It coordinates our interaction with the outside world, and adjusts our inner support system to this interaction: it is a coordinating and integrating unit that adapts our organism (mind and body) to outer and inner changes. It cools us down when the temperature inside or outside becomes too high, for example, and arranges our body into a sitting position when we want to sit down. If we drink too much water, the regulating system will remove the excess water through the kidneys. It generally tries to prevent any disturbances (entering our body from the outside world or happening accidentally inside the body) from becoming excessive, from going past certain safe limits.

It offers protection against invasion: we have a defensive system that has an intelligence and elimination unit.

It looks after healing (repair and maintenance) of normal wear and tear and of damage. This is a repair and maintenance unit.

Our practical emotional mind manages this regulating system as its highest manager at work. It sits in the driver's seat and controls the regulating system, and this is an important point to remember.

Everything that happens inside the living body must start with the emotional mind which must guide this body in its survival activities. This is similar to the principle that whatever a car on the road does is always the consequence of the driver's decisions, the only exception to this being an accident due to material fatigue.

The emotional and instinctive minds represent mother nature's attempts to keep the organism alive and active. We shall discuss regulation in a separate chapter and focus on defence in the rest of this chapter.

SELF-PROTECTION

One department of the self-protection system is a defensive system against any invasion of our body with foreign material, whether the invaders are alive or not. The defence systems are built into our body so that they work automatically; they are our internal defence systems.

Other methods of self-protection involve the organism itself by means of protective instincts and emotions; running or hiding from danger, looking for shelter from cold and rain, and special feeding and resting when ill. This self-protective system involves the emotional mind and represents a set of instructions for staying alive.

The human being has the advantage of a rational mind that can advise the emotional mind (if this will calm down enough and listen). The rational mind can invent improved and even new ways of self-protection, that the emotional mind can learn to use.

The internal protection department guards the body around the clock against invasion from the environment. Its detection system monitors the body just as a radar system scans the entire coastline of a country. When an invasion is reported by our detection (intelligence) system, this department quickly sends out elimination teams to get rid of the invader.

An invasion by material that is foreign to the body is called an infection. If the organism is to survive the invasion, this illegal entry must be detected, and the invader removed.

Two systems of defence: We have two systems of defence against infection.

(a) There is a general protection against any kind of invasion. This is called on first and this system is like a standing army that is more or less vigilant and ready to do battle. It is always on guard and primed to repel and eliminate invaders. This general system is our general inborn resistance against invasion, our natural immunity from invasion.

(b) There is also a special branch of the defence department that is made up of specially trained units that have the task of detecting and eliminating specific invaders. This system is a counter-insurgency unit that provides us with a specific and acquired immunity against enemy invasion. Here, the word acquired means: not built-in, but created through later contact.

Immunity from invasion and resistance against invasion mean the same thing: defence against invasion that is part of the larger and more general protection system. Protection from the environment means a rejection of any invasion of our organism by living or inanimate agents.

The efficiency of our general protective system depends on a number of factors. Some that influence the efficacy of our protective system, such as age, and genes, we cannot do anything about. But the emotional and rational minds together, have the important task of making sure that other conditions, such as rest, nutrition, proper treatment of illnesses, and freedom from stress, are properly attended to.

A stress-free and healthy emotional mind is of fundamental importance for natural self-protection, but nobody bothered to teach us that when we were children. We were too busy learning to do sums, and how to become stressed through ignorance and overwork.

There is normally a natural balance between our organism and the environment we live in. This natural environment is our natural habitat and we live in peace with it. But it can also become a potential invader. Let me explain:

This natural balance is a condition of relative peace between us and our environment. It is a working relationship of give and take. If this balance is disturbed by changes in the world or in us, then the state of peace is threatened, and may even be ended, unless our regulating system is capable of restoring it. Natural disasters, such as typhoons and epidemics, may threaten our well-being, but the peaceful balance can also be disturbed by stress in any form, such as illness, exhaustion, emotional stress. Stress reduces our self-protective strength against invasions.

We may state this in a shorter way by saying that we live in relative peace with the world. But this world is always ready to take advantage of any weakness that we may show, and invade our territory. In this disturbed balance, we may have to play the role of an unwilling host to some aggressive invader.

This balance means that the power of micro-organisms to invade our body is relative to our capacity for resistance (the power of our defence systems).

The more powerful our defence system is, the less dangerous our environment will be for us. A powerful defending army has less to fear from enemies than a weakened one. What may be a powerful enemy for a weak country, is merely an annoyance for another, and more powerful, country. The weaker the defending army is, the stronger the enemy will become in relation to it, so that even an ordinarily neutral environment may now become dangerous for a weakened organism.

It is important to realise that our organism is not usually at war with our environment. We mainly live in peaceful co-existence with the world of micro-organisms around us. We have a non-aggression pact with most of these. For as long as the normal conditions of life are maintained, this state of relative peace continues, but when our organism loses its full natural capacity for self-protection, this will cause some micro-organisms around us to become enemy agents, pressing to invade our body. They become the *pathogenic* invaders, we become the compromised or impaired host organism. Pathogenic means sick-making.

Our self-protective capacity is our host resistance. If this happens to be low for any reason (such as some illness, exhaustion, injury, poisoning, and emotional stress), it will automatically increase the invasive capacity of all micro-organisms. There is a delicate balance between our protective system and the aggressiveness of alien invaders. The healthier we are, the better we stand against these. The weaker we are, the more we are at risk. This aggressive capacity of micro-organisms for an invasion of our body is their virulence or malignancy.

In the case of cancer, the same balance applies. Cancer is an infection with abnormal material that has come from inside our own tissues. That should, ideally, be the only difference. Unfortunately, the degree of foreignness is not always so obvious that they can be detected very easily, particularly if the high level of alertness of our detection systems has been reduced by stress. Because they originate from normal parent-cells, some cancers may have ways of hiding from detection that are not yet fully understood.

Generally, however, the same balance applies: the healthier the host is in mind and body, the greater its self-protective power is. The greater this self-defending capacity is, the less dangerous the cancer cells will be, and vice versa. Stress is the most common and the most powerful suppressant of this protective system, because stress disorganises all our normal functions.

Stress means disorganisation: it is a disturbance that is too severe for our regulating system to cope with. It disorganises our total system, including body and mind. We can cope with mild noise, for example, and manage not to let it disturb our concentration or rest. A stronger noise, however, may be beyond our coping capacity, so that it distracts us from whatever we are trying to do. We are disorganised in our practical activity, we can't do anything because of the excessive noise, we feel frustrated, angry, and otherwise upset. We are stressed.

Stress and greater vulnerability to disease (disorder) go hand in hand.

We may normally expect our efficient body to behave towards cancer cells in the same self-protective manner as it resists invasion by micro-organisms. If it does not perform this task, we ask why not, and we look for factors that have reduced its normal efficiency. We ask questions:

What reduced its vigilance so that early cancer could escape detection by the quality-control unit? What has impaired the capacity of our organism to detect and remove such foreign material? And what can we, ourselves, do to restore it to good health?

We know from daily experience that resting in a stress-free environment, and proper nutrition, are of great importance in restoring the normal balance in illness and operations. This healing process is known as recuperation, and that means that the disorganised organism must be reorganised, restored to its normal well-being.

Our biological self-protective system has a powerful natural resistance against any kind of disturbance that may come our way to cause disorder in our orderly, functioning body. We have natural barriers against invasion, such as the skin and mucous membranes. We also possess natural buffering systems that act as shock absorbers. These work to cancel out any disturbance and injury.

If there is an invasion with material that is foreign to the body, then the detection and elimination systems (intelligence and army) begin their work quickly and efficiently. In one way or another, the harmful agent is detected and made harmless.

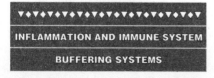

ENVIRONMENT

▼◆▼◆▼◆▼◆▼◆▼◆▼◆▼◆▼◆▼◆▼◆▼	= **NATURAL BARRIERS**
INFLAMMATION AND IMMUNE SYSTEM	= **DETECTION + ELIMINATION**
BUFFERING SYSTEMS	= **SHOCK ABSORBERS**

When these systems have completed their task, then the healing system is activated to perform repair and maintenance work and to do the cleaning up. The normal order of well-being is now restored.

The skin and mucous membranes that form the lining of the airways, bowels, and urinary system are natural barriers against invasion. Behind these barriers we find the army and intelligence departments. Behind army and intelligence systems we encounter the buffering systems, that also have the task of restoring the natural order. We may compare these to the fire brigade, ambulance, and other essential services.

Without such strong and effective natural defence systems, no life would be possible. What this also means is that we may take it for granted that the natural outcome of any infection, whether due to bacteria, viruses, parasites or cancer, will be a successful elimination of the danger, and a return to normal health. This also means that we should not neglect the important task of keeping ourselves in good condition.

We all depend on such successful recuperation in our everyday life, and we accept quite naturally that this happens, and that mother nature will protect us. We accept this in the same way that a baby takes it for granted that its mother will look after it. We also know that recovery works best when we cope with life, and that it does not work as well whenever we are stressed.

We have to do our bit also. We must contribute towards our own well-being because the state of good mental and bodily health is our best defence against illness.

There are a number of exceptional circumstances in medicine in which a person's natural defences are absent since birth, or have been deliberately suppressed by chemical agents, such as in organ transplantations. In these cases there is a constant fear of infection: infection with micro-organisms from the outside world, or a fear of cancer appearing.

We may accept that the natural outcome of infection is healing and if this does not happen, we must wake up and ask why not, and what we can do to assist mother nature in healing us. Sometimes healing does not happen spontaneously, at least not easily and immediately. We call this a complication of the infection, and we are often surprised by such a weakened state of our defence system. We did not expect it.

We then ask why such a complication had to appear, and we look for ways of restoring normal health. We may need to intervene, and assist our healing by resting in freedom from stress, by attending to proper nutrition and, if necessary, by medication and surgery.

A complication means that something has gone wrong with normal healing, and we look for the disturbing agent that has sapped power from the healing and defence systems. We may find this disturbance located in the body (malnutrition, other illness, exhaustion) or in the emotional mind as emotional stress or, more usually, as a combination of both physical and emotional (psychological) stress.

The development of clinical cancer from the early infection with cancer cells is a complication that should normally not have occurred. When we ask why this complication came about, we usually come up with the main and most common suppressive agent: stress.

Stress is more than just having a difficult time. We have a coping system to deal with that. Stress means that we are no longer coping, and that our system is no longer capable of regulating the disturbance, whatever it may be (physical or psychological).

Our emotional mind digests experience in a way that is often comparable to the manner in which our digestive system deals with food. Over-eating or a heavy meal requires a greater effort from our stomach so that it takes longer to digest, but this is not indigestion; a sound stomach can cope with the greater load by working harder, but it is not stressed.

Indigestion appears if we eat something that is indigestible for this digestive system. It becomes frustrated in its efforts, and may break down in its attempts to deal with the problem. The consequence of this failure to digest the indigestible lump is a blocked stomach, first with vomiting and painful cramps, and later with paralysis, as if it is now resigned to the impossibility of dealing with the problem. That is stress.

Stress indicates failure. Our system is now disorganised in all its workings. Our organism is in disarray and disorder, so that nothing works properly (effectively) any more. Our body can now only fail to protect and regulate itself.

Stress is often the cause of complications that may arise during and after surgery. But this has not been sufficiently recognised.

The illness itself, as well as the family, work, and economic problems that come with it, are stress factors that only add to the trauma of the operation and anaesthetic. Patients undergo operations without any preparation in stress management. Yet they are expected to have their proper routine physical pre-operative checkup. Doctors always listen to their hearts and lungs, but never to their minds. Are we still so blind to the needs of the besieged emotional mind?

Stress suppresses effective detection, removal, and healing, simply by disorganising these vitally important functions. Instead of recuperating, patients develop complications.

We usually depend on rest, nutrition, and medication and even surgery to assist defence and healing, but sometimes this is not enough, and we must add another way of helping nature. This is called psychological intervention. It means that we must correct a wrong emotional mindset that has been interfering with our well-being and, therefore, with proper healing.

The healing of the emotional mind is of utmost importance for the healing of the body, and we discuss the reason for saying this later in part three.

IMMUNE SURVEILLANCE

Sir Macfarlane Burnet wrote a book on immunology and called it, significantly, *Self and NOT-Self*. In this book he offers the idea of the possible existence of an immune surveillance team: a surveillance system that is newer, and more sophisticated, than the older unit which deals with the more basic inflammatory responses.

Although this surveillance theory, as he proposed it, has not been generally accepted, the notion of a surveillance system makes good biological sense, and fits in well with what we know about the biology of defence.

According to the modified immune surveillance theory, which has gained considerable popularity among immunologists, it is quite possible that the body will produce cancer cells now and then as replacement and repair goes on.

We know that the entire body renews itself every few months, with bone tissue taking longest to be renewed. From sheer probability alone, we may already expect that sooner or later some cells will derail from their normal division, and become cancerous, possibly assisted by abnormal conditions. This idea is supported by the fact that cancer is most often seen in those active tissues that have the greatest turnover of cells. These are the tissues that are most directly involved in interchange with our environment. They are, as we said earlier, mainly the normal protective coverings of our body (skin and mucous membranes) that form our front-line barriers to invasion, and gland tissue.

Although we now assume that anybody can develop cancer cells in their body, not everyone develops clinical cancer, which means: established cancer. Why not? Because the keen surveillance system detects their presence, and has them destroyed immediately. This is what we called in a previous chapter quality control at their birth.

In a minority of cases this does not happen naturally. There may be a number of reasons for this:

(a) Oncological reasons that have to do with the qualities of the tumour tissue itself.

(b) Age plays a role; older people usually have less effective defensive systems.

(c) Stress (physical or psychological) interferes with normal surveillance. Illness, exhaustion, malnutrition, emotional stress, are all important resistance lowering factors. This aspect is the main focus of this book.

TRIBAL LAWS OF THE BODY

Our body tissues are bound by very primitive tribal laws that make them suspicious and intolerant of any foreign material in their midst. Cancer is not welcome; its presence is normally as little tolerated as that of any other foreign substance. This is a strict law of nature. We see it in bacterial communities and animals as well as in humans.

Our normal skin and bowel bacteria remove any foreign bacteria that happen to invade their territory, for example, paying for their tolerated housing on our surfaces in that way.

Animals are defensive about their own territory, so that these are hostile environments for foreign invaders. Few human communities will tolerate foreign-looking strangers as well as they accept their own kind. This tribal attitude is still very strong in us. In older days, strangers were usually either killed or taken captive. They were rarely welcomed.

A healthy body is extremely intolerant of foreign material because this is practical strategy, important for survival. While we should try to overcome this intolerance on a social level by understanding that we belong to the same human species, we should allow the body to be as rigidly intolerant as possible, when it concerns foreign invasion, from chemicals to cancer.

The question that we should ask is perhaps not: 'How is it possible that the cancer manages to survive and grow?' We should perhaps ask more directly: 'What has happened to our defences? How is it possible that they are so suppressed that the cancer escapes detection and elimination?'

This question shifts our attention to the weakness and failure of effective detection and removal rather than looking for certain qualities that the cancer cells themselves may have, which would explain how they manage to survive inside us.

The body is designed to be practical, which means to survive, and often against great odds. All our tissues have practical work to perform. Our tonsils and appendix were long thought to be unnecessary and useless tissues, but we know now that they have a defensive function, they form an important part of our total defensive system. They are no longer routinely removed.

This also means that anything that has no practical use in the body will be removed by our immune defences. Only malformations are tolerated in their uselessness. They are not part of our normal design, but their cells are basically our own, even if they are not in their normal place. We could describe it as normal useless tissue.

Cancer is an example of abnormal useless tissue. By rights it should be quickly eliminated from the body. We may expect that this usually happens; cancer is usually eliminated as soon as it is detected. In certain cases this evidently does not happen, so that such early cancer grows into a clinically detectable cancer that causes symptoms of its presence. This is clinical cancer.

This is a situation that we are familiar with from other kinds of infection. We call this a complication of the infection. Why? Because we normally expect, and even take it for granted, that any infection can be overcome and made to disappear from the body. And clinical cancer is a complication of early cancer.

We do not normally expect meningitis to complicate a sore throat or measles, or suspect peritonitis or a liver abscess with appendicitis. We are merely aware of the possibility that this may happen if the resistance of the host organism is not up to its normal level. Complications are not part of the normal course of infections.

Psychosomatic research has shown that there are reasons for reduced resistance which are not inside the organism, but exist in a disturbed emotional relationship between the person and the world. Physical factors can reduce our vital host resistance, and emotional ones are equally important. These do their harmful work through emotional stress.

DETECTION OF DIFFERENCES

The key notion in the detection of any infection is that there is always a difference between what is self, and what is not-self in the body. This difference can be recognised. Invaders belong to the not-self. Finding the difference is therefore the task of both our intelligence systems that work, or should work, around the clock. Identifying the not-self is the first step in its rejection. Stress dopes our intelligence system by severely disorganising its efficiency in identifying our enemies!

This detection of differences between self and not-self is also of great importance in our psychological development from child to adult. During this development we learn to separate all that is emotionally self, from all which is not-self; from the world which does not belong to the self. This separation is a rejection of the not-self. Only when the child recognises its own existence does it also recognise the existence of the other, the not-self, the you. When the child learns to say 'I', it has, at the same time, learnt to say no and you. The term 'I' means: not-you, and what you really mean is: all that is not-me.

The child that is not yet capable of making this distinction between self and not-self, is very vulnerable because it will accept suggestions from others as if these were its own. Its emotional mind cannot tell the difference between what comes from itself and what originated with others. The child is therefore highly suggestible, and open to bad influences. This may well be regarded as an emotional infection: an infection of a defenceless emotional mind.

We may be capable of a critical rejection of something by our rational mind, but we are not so clearly aware and resistant on the emotional level. We absorb feelings and make them our own, while our rational mind rejects them on rational grounds.

We return to this stage whenever we are emotionally upset; in other words, stressed. We become abnormally suggestible, and then we can swallow, without any mental resistance, the myth that cancer is an inevitable death sentence. We can snort at this ridiculous idea if we ourselves don't have cancer, but we become vulnerable to this myth if we do. No matter how much our rational mind may protest, our emotional mind doesn't listen. The rational mind is now no longer heard. It has been moved to the back seat of our organism. Whenever our emotions are strong, we run hot and our rational mind becomes silent.

Our first and foremost defence against emotional infection is not the activity of our rational mind, but above all, relaxation; this calms the emotional mind and makes it open to reason, receptive to advice by the rational mind. This is how we manage to reject the voodoo myth.

This myth is like a malignant computer virus that infects our normal programs. It is a psychological cancer that invades our emotional mind without much resistance, and grows there to do its bad work, causing us to die an unnecessary voodoo death.

The intelligence system of the body must be able to recognise its own tissues, to recognise the different organs and cells inside itself. It must also be able to perceive the world that belongs to the not-self, and tell the difference between this not-self and self. At every moment of our life we must make continual distinctions between self and not-self, or we could not perceive anything or do anything. We could not function as living beings. Making emotional distinctions and detecting organic differences are functions of our protective system. Defence of our emotional mind is just as important as that of our body.

All our life processes depend on making such distinctions, and on maintaining these differences. Our internal intelligence must be able to tell the heart from the brain and the joints from the muscles. It must also be able to detect the presence of foreign material, so that this notion of surveillance is in line with all other biological functions.

As far as our normally functioning body is concerned, it cannot afford to be tolerant of foreigners, and it has to remain primitive, tribal. The tribal law of primitive societies says: kill that foreigner now or make a slave out of him. A foreigner is a foe, and never wait to prove otherwise.

The living body is surrounded by potential foes, and must always remain totally ruthlessly tribal to survive. It cannot afford to slacken its vital intelligence work against possible invasion, and it cannot afford to be soft against any cancer cells. It must not accept the cancer as part of the family.

The ability to tell the difference between self and not-self, and to reject all that is not-self, is severely impaired in stress. This disorganisation happens not only to the body, but also to the emotional mind. Such disarray will show up in both body and mind. An example:

Mr TCP has cancer. The ruthless defence system of his body has been impaired, his body has failed to reject the cancer cells. Does his emotional mind do better? To test this, we shall now ask him to visualise the cancer cells, to recognise them as outlaws that do not belong in his normal body, and to imagine that he must remove them. How does he visualise doing this? He picks them up and puts them in the rubbish bin, or chases them away with a broom.

No, we tell him, that's a pretty weak gesture, Mr TCP.

Don't be so civilised, imagine that you are your intolerant body; take a big hammer and squash them, or grind them under your heel. Be completely ruthless in your dealings with these baddies! He tries again, but he can't do it.

Mr TCP can't do it, he cannot bring himself to be ruthless even to save himself, and that is quite characteristic for the quality of his emotional resistance to life's problems.

An immune-suppressed body cannot recognise a foreign invader with normal efficiency, so it can't fight back properly. It is severely compromised, and endangered. A stressed mind can no longer tell the difference between what belongs to the self and what is not-self as sharply as before the stress. It is less efficient, and loses track of the difference between 'you' and 'me'.

This is a regressive symptom that is known as identification or participation, and means that the organism has become more primitive; it has lost its sophisticated capacity to discern fine differences between self and not-self.

The lines that this mind has earlier learned to draw between self and not-self have become blurred, so that it becomes open to outside suggestions, to brain-washing, and to other foreign influences; open to emotional infection.

This also applies to the body; its ability to discriminate and to reject is compromised, so that it may fail to distinguish between cancer cell and normal body cells.

The more abnormal cancer cells become, the more they change towards the not-self, so that they no longer belong to our normal body. They have now become *antigenic*: capable of provoking a total rejection.

If this recognition of their otherness does not take place, it is a failure of regulation. Something must have gone wrong with the efficiency of recognition, and this something is usually the immune-suppressant effect of stress; physical, chemical, or emotional.

Imagine that you have scratched yourself on a dirty thorn in the garden. If your defensive system is functioning properly, the invasion with bacteria will be detected, so that a proper inflammatory response is under way within six to eight hours.

The response may be mild in the case of a scratch, and the signs of swelling, redness, heat, and pain, usually disappear in a few days, so that everything is back to normal, and you can use the part normally again.

This is the natural course of any invasion, or no life would be possible. It means that we may, and should, always expect healing to take place. And if it does not, we must ask why not.

There is no reason not to expect this to happen in cases of cancer. If accidentally produced cancer cells grow out into clinical cancer, we must ask: what went wrong? Something must have happened to interfere seriously with the normal workings of the practical and efficient protection system. Where and what is the cause of this regulation failure?

Traditional physical medicine looks for physical causes of trouble, such as viruses, chemical irritants, and radiation. Psychosomatic medicine asks: is the emotional mind involved in this problem? This is not at all a stupid question when we now realise that our life runs on emotional programmes, and that it is primarily ruled by emotional logic. Everything that happens in the body, we say, begins in the emotional mind. The exception to this, as we said in another context, is an accident which is due to material weakness or fatigue.

For example: Someone, let us say, a Ms Unlucky, has developed AIDS. We say that it is the HIV virus that causes AIDS. But is this enough? Shouldn't we also ask where it began? Why she got into a situation which exposed her to this infection? At the origin of this story lies the unfortunate emotional decision to have intercourse with someone, a carrier whom she obviously did not know well enough or who did not care enough to safeguard her. What motivated her to do this?

As with any other kind of illness, AIDS has different levels of causation: at the highest and most general level, which is that of behaviour and its motivation, we have the emotional mind. At the lowest level, we have more mechanical causes of cell disturbance (a virus, genetic accident or poison).

Another example: A child catches a cold. What causes colds? Some cold virus, of course. And what else? Let us trace this cause back from the virus to the conduct of the organism: the virus is transmitted, in this case, by droplet infection. Someone sneezed or coughed near the child, and the child inhaled an infected droplet of mucus. The child was at school and it was winter time, so that the classroom doors and windows were closed. This is how infected air keeps circulating throughout the whole classroom.

Is this all? Not yet, because we still have to ask why this child developed the cold, and why his five other friends, who were equally exposed, did not get it. What was wrong with his defensive system? Why did it not protect this child?

Was he malnourished, ill with something else, exhausted? Was he suffering from anything else that could have reduced normal resistance, such as emotional stress? Why was the child who spread the cold sent to school by his parents?

We usually end up with motives, with involvement on the level of the emotional mind, when we care to trace such infections back to their root. A virus is only the mechanical part of the chain of events that lead to a viral illness.

Emotions are not at all those things that are described in the usual textbooks of psychology and psychiatry. Emotions are processes inside the body as well as entire programs for living – more like complex software programs that direct the entire computer system.

These affect the entire organism, because they must guide this system in its survival behaviour. They will determine (or at least influence) whatever goes on inside the body. That is why they are so important in all aspects of psychosomatic medicine. In short, we don't have emotions, they have us, they guide us, they control our organism. We, as our rational mind, can have control over the emotional mind – which means that it will listen to reason – only when the emotions are so weak that they no longer overwhelm us.

Our rational mind is the rational part of our personality that can think theoretically, ask questions and discuss with others what it thinks.

Feelings, including all emotions and sensations, form the software, the vital guiding instructions that run our organism and must guarantee its survival. A feeling is not merely one single thing, like a word or a picture: every feeling is a complete programme for behaviour. It is a complete but condensed short story. If a picture is worth a thousand words, then one feeling is equal to a thousand pictures. Our rational mind may be too slow to read the feeling, but our body computer does it in a flash.

Stress, because it always contains abnormal (disorganising) feelings, will both delay detection and reduce the functions of defence and healing, so that the infection is more severe than it needs to be. Stress weakens our system, and makes it more vulnerable to invasion.

This is a very important point. The aggressive and sick-making capacity of micro-organisms, and of cancer cells, is never an absolute factor. It is relative to the defensive capacity of the host. This relation is therefore a see-saw relationship: the stronger the host, the weaker the invading organism. The reverse is: the weaker the host, the stronger the invader.

The strength of the human host that is being invaded, depends on its physical and emotional well-being. When we use the word 'mind', we generally employ it to indicate both the rational (intellectual) and emotional minds. We only separate them so clearly for the sake of an easier understanding. It is the emotional mind that is involved in our well-being, and we shall use the word mind for the emotional mind unless the intellectual mind is mentioned by name.

If you are host to an infection with bacteria, viruses, or cancer, and you are not sick or stressed, then you may well assume that you will heal, because your defensive and healing systems are working normally: practically and powerfully. Healing is the rule, and we take this for granted in our everyday life. If a complication should arise, so that the infection becomes a clinically detectable infection, then something has probably gone wrong with your normal defences.

If you are suffering from stress, then these functions, like all other functions of your body and mind, are in a state of disorganisation. You feel weary and irritable, you can't think straight, you can't concentrate well, you may have diarrhoea, stomach discomfort, headaches, you may also feel anxious and restless, can't sleep, and your resistance against infections is low.

When we are not stressed, we should feel fit. The symptoms of normal practical living are the feelings of fitness and well-being. Most of our actions are then also practical: useful for survival in some way.

When we suffer from stress, this sense of practical fitness in well-being is lost, and we have other feelings that are no longer practical instructions for living, such as nervousness, unease, anger, anxiety, weariness, irritability or depression. All that such abnormal feelings can now be useful for, is to make us aware of their presence, as indicators that all is not well with us. Apart from this, they are entirely worthless.

There is a whole supermarketful of possible stress symptoms. But they all mean one thing: they are totally useless for an organism that is born to be practical. Poor self-image has as little meaning as a bout of diarrhoea or a nervous cough. It is equally impractical: these are merely useless stress symptoms. Only in exceptional cases do we need to look for some symbolic significance in such stress symptoms.

There is rarely any need to analyse such stress feelings. You have them only because you are stressed, and you can get rid of them by systematic relaxation instead. When the stress is gone, the symptoms usually disappear. We do not have to drag in the past to explain them and deal with them. Only if they have not faded spontaneously, do we need to search out the past for problems that began in the past, and that have remained active in the present, where they may express themselves in a symbolic form.

Under stress, nothing can work properly; our organism is in a state of relative malfunctioning, it is disorganised, so that it is no longer organised for practical living. We have functions that keep our organism working properly, our so called regulating systems, and when these fail under stress we begin to feel unbalanced, unfit, uneasy, and unwell.

We shall look at these regulating systems in chapter eight.

Chapter Seven

HOST RESISTANCE

One of the first lectures on the pathology of infections in medical school is usually a talk on the relationship between an invading micro-organism and the host, the body that has been invaded. The micro-organism tries to invade our body, and our body resists.

Invasion and resistance determine each other, and one cannot be understood without considering the other. Normally, the host is capable of resisting the advances of any potential invader. If it is invaded, it has the power to overcome the enemy and restore the normal order. This is how the organism has been designed to perform.

As we have seen, this relation depends on the ability of the body to tell what belongs to its 'self', and what is not part of itself, and to keep the two apart. It performs this task in much the same way that a country guards its borders against unauthorised entry by aliens; it uses a system of passport checking.

It is also the way in which a little child learns to say 'you' to anything that does not belong to itself, to 'me'. It learns to keep self and not-self separate in its emotional mind in the same way in which its body does that. As it experiences the world around itself, a living organism must automatically separate all that is not-self from the self.

We shall try to show that it does not matter to the passport-checking body whether the invader is a thorn, a bacterium or a cancer cell, as long as this body is in good enough shape to recognise a foreign passport, so that the foreigner can be unconditionally and totally rejected. It must be able to tell the difference between that foreign passport, and the passport that its own citizens have, and for this task our organism must be fit and free of stress.

Such a passport is made up of the specific immune-spectrum of tissue proteins. Foreign tissue has qualities that differ from the body's own tissues, and if an alert passport-checking body finds that the two do not match, then this invader with its foreign passport will be rejected without further ado.

The foreign passport of invaders is their antigenic quality, and this antigenic quality has two effects on the body:

(a) It marks the invader as being an unwanted alien.

(b) Once this alien invader has been so marked, the defensive systems of the body are activated for its speedy removal.

This body must be in a condition of emotional and physical well-being, if it is to be alert and vigilant. After all, we cannot expect our customs officers to be watchful if they are ill or depressed.

They are more likely to make mistakes under stress, and let in criminals that will then try to take over the country. The significance of stress as an immune suppressant is now an important issue in the studies of biological immunity.

Micro-organisms that invade the body, can cause harm in four ways:

   (i) by invading aggressively;

  (ii) by multiplying quickly;

 (iii) by producing harmful substances (toxins);

 (iv) by producing treatment-resistant forms;

These four factors determine the virulence of invading micro-organisms which is their capacity for harming the host organism.

The degree of malignancy (this means the same as virulence) of tumour cells depends on exactly the same four factors:

   (i) their invasive capacity;

  (ii) their ability to multiply quickly;

 (iii) tumours may produce substances that hamper resistance;

 (iv) their ability to breed treatment-resistant forms.

Cancer cells and micro-organisms are antigenic; their tissue is so different from that of the host, that their foreign presence can be detected, and a defensive response can be called up. Our entire defence system is based on the capacity of our intelligence systems to detect the presence of foreign material; everything that is not-self, not part of our own body.

If the host organism is in a state of physical and emotional well-being, then this healthy organism should treat cancer as it would any other infection: detect, attack, overcome, and heal.

How powerful are our defence and healing systems? This question may be answered with another question: how many living beings are there in the world? If these systems were not strong enough, there would be no life on earth, not even the most primitive of organisms would be capable of surviving.

Life depends on the capacity of the body for self-protection: for effective defence and healing. This is the most basic program for surviving. Defence is based on the recognition of danger and its removal. Healing is the capacity of the organism to repair itself, and to make itself whole again.

Lower organisms have the amazing ability to grow back certain parts of the body that have been lost. While as higher human organisms we can no longer do that, our powers of restitution are still considerable.

This means that we must accept that the normal course of any infection is such, that it must end in healing.

Virulence, which is the capacity of the invader to do harm, is normally cancelled out by resistance, which is the capacity of the host to defend itself against any kind of illness, and to heal itself. This is a see-saw arrangement: the stronger the host, the less virulent the invader, and vice versa.

The same is true for cancer; the weaker the host, the more malignant the cancer and vice versa. This means that we should do all that we can to avoid weakening our natural resistance, and do everything possible to improve it.

Effective host resistance depends, not only on the well-being of the body, but equally on our emotional well-being, on our emotional fitness for living. Everything that happens inside our body is ultimately influenced by this. The old saying of 'a healthy mind inside a healthy body' should be reversed; a healthy body inside a healthy mind.

While this may sound strange to more old-fashioned doctors, it appears quite natural to a psychosomatically inclined modern medical person. Psychosomatic medicine is full of examples which demonstrate the powerful effect that our emotional state can have on the see-saw arrangement between invader virulence and host resistance.

A telling anecdote about a German professor of hygiene in the last century (Max von Pettenkofer) relates how, during a medical conference, he was listening with growing impatience to a still young Dr Koch discussing his experiments with cholera bacteria. Koch had proved that the tiny germs were the cause of this serious disease.

As Dr Koch showed the audience a tube containing a culture of virulent cholera bacteria, the sceptical Professor von Pettenkofer took the test tube out of Koch's hand and drank the contents, to prove that this was just nonsense. And what happened to him? Nothing. The man simply refused to believe that there could be even a possibility that a little creature like that, invisible to the naked eye, was the cause of something as bad as cholera. Becoming sick was not an option. The possibility probably did not occur to him.

There have been many other attempts to explain his immunity, such as having had too much acid in his empty stomach when he drank it, but this is looking for the answer in the wrong place. It was simply not possible that he could get sick from drinking the culture, because he was convinced that it was nonsense.

A conviction, which is an unshakeable belief, has a powerful organising or dis-organising influence on our system. Strong beliefs are based on intense emotions, and intense feelings, if they are normal, have the biological task of organising our system for its practical activities: for survival.

An intense positive emotion is a strong organising force; it concentrates our system in the direction of that feeling, and this is either action or healing.

An equally intense, but negative emotion, can disorganise us with the same power, so that our system is in a condition of disarray: it is no longer organised and working to stay alive. A strong fear organises our system into becoming an efficient running machine; when danger threatens, we run fast to safety. A panic attack, on the other hand, dis-organises us totally, so that we have a sense of unreality and utter helplessness. We are paralysed and good for nothing.

A voodoo death is an example of such complete disintegration resulting from a wrong belief; such wrong beliefs are supported by intense and abnormal emotions.

Intense positive beliefs contain emotions that stimulate the life impulse in us, which concentrate it, so to speak. The intense positive belief brings this life impulse to new heights of organisation, so that we become capable of feats of action or healing that are not generally required in our ordinary course of living.

We have a reserve capacity for maintaining life that we rarely need to call on. This extra capacity becomes accessible only through intense (voluntary or involuntary) concentration, and it is usually only open to us in extra-ordinary (non-ordinary) circumstances.

The important will to live has nothing to do with a voluntary decision of our rational mind: this 'will' is a profound need or urge to continue life, it is a belief in the worth of being (and staying) alive; it is a determination to heal and live.

A new-found love, for example, can fire up this will to live, and we may regard this as a strongly focused concentration on living. Such strong beliefs can reverse the wrong direction of illness.

The central factor in all intense emotions and strong beliefs is simply the degree of concentration of our attention on the topic. Strong feelings concentrate our attention involuntarily and we refer to this state when we say that we are fascinated, spellbound, charmed, preoccupied, obsessed, compelled, and so on. Feelings are natural hypnosis-producing phenomena.

Concentration, we may say, is the 'lens' of the creative life force in us. When the lens contracts, it magnifies this life impulse, and if we slacken this lens, we disperse and reduce the strength of this biological energy.

We can relax or make monotonous rhythmic movements to produce a concentrated state of our attention by voluntary means. Having achieved this concentrated state, we then devote intense attention to the topic for a while. We visualise the effect that we wish to achieve.

Most, if not all, ancient religions have developed such a concentration method. This involves making rhythmic movements with the body and this is intensified by singing the prayer in the same rhythm. Singing and moving with the song have been used since the early days of humankind in prayer and lullaby to settle the emotional mind. This allows it to concentrate on other things or to simply rest a while.

We rarely need this degree of concentration of attention in our ordinary daily routine, where we make use of a scanning kind of attention that searches out the world around us.

These feats of action and healing are not mysterious powers, simply non-ordinary tasks that require special attentive devotion and learning. Houdini used the trick of swallowing the key to the locks and, like a yogi, bringing it up again when he needed it.

Strong beliefs may bring us to unusual heights of resistance and healing if they are positive, or cause a rapid deterioration if negative. Positive strong beliefs can open the future for our organism, negative ones may close it.

Stress may involve us with strongly negative feelings. If it endures and is severe, such stress can become a damper on the life impulse in us. It narrows our access to the future, and this reduces our resistance to illness. The degree of stress that we call demoralisation, may close off this path to the future; it can block the stream of life.

Our living organism is strongly influenced by our emotional mind, both in its well-being and in its illness.

HOW MIND AND BODY RELATE

The emotional mind guides the body in all its functions, and it does this either directly, such as stiffening up the muscles in tension, or indirectly, such as when it produces symptoms of disorganisation in stress, for example, palpitations or diarrhoea.

Let us imagine this situation more clearly. We usually think of the mind as being somewhere inside the body; in Western countries, the seat of the mind is supposed to be the head or brain, whereas in other traditions it is often assumed that it is located in the stomach, the liver or the heart. The notion that the mind exists somewhere inside the body is only a mechanistic way of thinking. It is now outdated.

The mind, according to phenomenological research, is not in the body. The reality is exactly the reverse: the body is in the mind, but not in a mechanistic way, not located in any space (see chapter thirty-one for more detail). The body is embraced by the mind, it is that part of the mind which has taken on form, simply because it has to carry out routine, relatively unchanging, practical work. The body is the part of the mind that has taken on the appearance of a structure so that it can do its habitual repetitive work.

We would never use the wind for a fence, for example, because we want the fence to continue to do its work of fencing off the garden: we would not want it to change itself. On the other hand, we would not use a fence for producing a cool breeze, or for making music: we can't feel the passing of a flowing fence (we would not wish to), nor can we hear a fence as a melody, or as a wave of anger. The less changeable the work (function) has to be, the more it becomes a formed and stable structure.

The mind makes use of the body in the same way that any software programme makes use of its hardware (which is the machine, as a fixed and unchanging structure) to display itself. The hardware represents that part of the software that does not need to change. Our emotional mind uses its body for its routine work. We may state this differently: the body is the routine working part of the mind.

Imagine that you are a cleaner, and that you must clean a room regularly. First, you do it in a very primitive way by wetting your hands in a nearby river, then you clean a little area of the room with these wet hands, then run quickly back to the river to clean and wet them. You do this repeatedly. After a while, you think of more effective ways of doing the job. You invent a bucket to hold a larger volume of water, a cloth to do the cleaning, a broom for sweeping, and so on. You begin to use things, instruments, for those parts of the job that always have to be done in the same way. This is how the emotional mind uses the body: as hardware for the routine and repetitive parts of the job of survival, as a convenient structure.

Without programs, what could we do with a computer? A TV is not a TV if there is nothing to display: it is a piece of junk. The machinery is only part of the whole system of writers, producers, sound engineers, editors, and so on.

This idea is not so strange; you only need to look at someone doing something to realise that what you are looking at is the mind in action, the mind using the body for its practical work, and that this body is only part of the story of this action.

Host resistance is in the first place an emotional (mental) resistance. What happens inside the body in terms of inflammation or immune defence is ultimately part and parcel of emotional behaviour. The emotional mind organises, and the body acts out the instructions.

Someone, for example, is very sensitive to cold air, especially night air, and must throw a scarf around his throat, or else suffer a heavy cold. He has experienced again and again that this happens, so it is not just imagination. He does get sick, and then usually has to stay home for a day or two.

One night, though, he had an intense disagreement with his wife about some people at a dinner party they had to go to. He felt so rebellious that he recklessly refused to put something warm around his neck, or even a coat, although it was winter. With only a shirt on and with an open neck at that, he went into the dark and cold night. And nothing happened to him; his anger simply made it impossible for him to catch a cold, in the same way that von Pettenkofer did not develop cholera.

How do we understand this? In the state of anger, his mind was narrowed on the focus of this anger, and there was no room for anything else, so catching a cold was now not even an option. It is not merely that the thought never entered his mind, but the very possibility of catching a cold was not open to him in the fully concentrated condition of his emotional mind on the angry topic. The risk was simply not there.

All psychosomatic phenomena are based on this totally intense concentration of the emotional mind on some focal point. This includes hypnosis, hysterical state, relaxation, and religious fervour. All the miracles of achievement in these mental states are based on this ability for total focusing of the emotional mind. What it focuses on is a feeling or belief that becomes a conviction, a certainty. There is no other option available; nothing else can happen.

This ability is shared by everybody as an involuntary effect of strong emotions, but it must be learned as a voluntary way of influencing the body.

General practice is full of such examples. More than half of it consists of psychosomatic medicine in one form or another. Some people say that they are too busy to get sick during an influenza epidemic. They say that they cannot afford to get sick. And they don't get sick or, at least, not easily, and not severely. Such resistance shows that a virus alone is not enough to cause illness.

Other people fall ill from emotional motives, and this means: stress. Children under stress (they are usually highly sensitive children) can be sick every second week. Such catarrhal children have been intensively investigated, and nothing abnormal has been found in the body.

Nothing abnormal usually means: 'There is nothing wrong with you', implying that it is all due to imagination. As if there was nothing wrong with a powerful, but wrongly working, imagination under stress.

The more sensitive people are (even in childhood), the more prone they will be to suffering from stress.

The emotional mind needs the body for practical living, for displaying itself in that practical manner that we call surviving, or staying alive and well. But it may also use the body to express wrong emotional instructions (such as unhappiness) by becoming sick or by dying. This can only happen if there is no option, no other way out.

The emotional mind then becomes totally focused on this wrong instruction as the only way, and becomes convinced of it. We may recognise the state of mind that Mr TCP is in, and realise that he has a serious disorder of the emotional mind, a demoralised condition that requires urgent treatment. This demoralised state is a mind set, focused on dying. Surviving is no longer an option.

Lowered resistance may have its emotional root. It may be an emotional issue before it becomes a bodily problem, and if we keep this in mind, we shall not forget to ask what emotional situation we are in, whenever we become ill.

STRESS AND RESISTANCE

Stress and resistance have a see-saw relationship. When stress goes up, resistance comes down. And when stress comes down, as we have said, resistance goes up. We know what resistance is: it is the natural capacity of the organism to defend itself against invasion, and to heal from it.

But what is stress? As long as you don't start thinking about it, it seems so obvious. And the great problem in research is: if you don't really know when normal working tension becomes stress, or if there is a difference between tension and stress, how are you then going to find out how people react to stress, and how stress relates to the growth of cancer?

As we can see, stress reduces resistance; it works against us, and works for disorder, for cancer and for any other kind of alien invasion (infection). Stress, whatever its origin, always disorganises our practically organised system.

Stress, in daily human life, is almost always emotional stress, meaning that we may find ourselves trapped in a situation that is too difficult for us to cope with, in an impossible situation. This, as we shall see, is entrapment.

Stress is coping failure. It is a disorganised condition of our practically organised system that is geared to survival. We shall see, in the chapters that follow, what stress means, and what coping failure implies.

Stress lowers our resistance against any invasion. This refers to invasion of the body as well as that of the emotional mind. It thus lowers our resistance against 'enemy propaganda', so that it makes us more open for wrong beliefs that may produce a malignant mindset. This faulty mindset is a psychological cancer.

Reducing stress means restoring the natural resistance of the body and mind. Escape from entrapment means: re-moralisation, renewed hope, and a proper fighting spirit for an organism that is born to cope. It allows us to produce the right beliefs that produce an effective mindset.

It means re-orienting and re-focusing the mind on health and well-being.

What about these right beliefs? We shall have to ask questions such as: 'Am I not really kidding myself with such 'positive' stuff? What is the truth about the outcome of this cancer, and my chances for the future?' That will be the subject of Part Four of this book.

Chapter Eight

REGULATION SYSTEMS

EMOTIONAL MIND AS DIRECTOR		
NERVOUS SYSTEM AS MANAGER		
ACTION SYSTEM	ACTION SUPPORT SYSTEM	LIFE-SUPPORT SYSTEM • Protection • Healing

The world of the senses that we live in, is our natural habitat. It is the playground of life, from which we must take our nourishment. At the same time, it is a potentially dangerous environment from which we must protect ourselves.

The phenomenon of life is a very orderly and highly complex organisation of functions that are geared to self-maintenance.

Everything in this system is controlled by rules and regulations: by strict life-sustaining protocols. Any intrusion by disorder into this carefully regulated system works as a disturbance of the life order, and it must be quickly and effectively removed or, if such elimination is not possible, at least be made harmless.

If you stir a quiet pond, you create a disturbance in it, but this settles after a while, because natural laws return it to its original condition, unless the disturbance is so great that the pond stays disturbed, or takes on a different form of order.

Living systems do not depend on such natural laws to even out disturbances. They have a specialised system which has the task of cancelling irregularities so that disorder ceases and normal order returns. This is our regulating system.

The nervous system regulates and supervises the body in action and it has a special branch that regulates the support systems for this action function (the autonomic nervous system). Our nervous system is a regulating system and works like an efficient general manager who must make sure that everything runs smoothly, and on time. Part of this nervous system is a special regulating department which has a vital task to fulfil: a life-support system of defence and healing. This system has the task of safeguarding our normal health and well-being.

This life-support regulating system usually manages to keep us fit and fine-tuned, balanced and healthy, by regular internal servicing. It does this when we periodically rest from our activity. We rest so that we may undergo a major internal service, just as a car must have its engine switched off and cooled before the mechanics can begin their work of repair and maintenance.

Organisms that can actively move around are such complicated systems that they need regular servicing even if they don't seem to have to rest to be serviced. Lower organisms may be able to service themselves even while they move around, but mobile systems of a higher order must switch off their engine, in order to undergo proper repair and maintenance.

Living beings have a self-servicing system that is designed to ensure the body performs smoothly and effectively:

(a) It provides the working body with enough fuel and oxygen (energy) for its activities. This is a supportive function of the self-servicing system, an action-support system.

(b) It protects the body from too much disturbance. Disturbance is anything that might upset the body, such as an infection, or trauma by physical, chemical or emotional agents, or an internal accident. This is its protective function:

(i) to resist any disturbance and to prevent it from entering;

(ii) to cancel out the disturbance if it does enter the system;

(iii) to restore the normal order after dealing with it.

(c) It heals any damage caused by the disturbance. This is its restorative or recuperative function: it restores the body to a state of well-being, it does repair and maintenance work.

The functions under (b) and (c) together form a vital life-support system.

All these functions taken together are called regulation, and what is being regulated is the emotional and bodily well-being of the organism, so that it can keep going and surviving.

In higher forms of life, we see a natural cycle of alternate activity and rest. The organism must rest for recuperation, it must cease its activity before repair can begin. While this organism is at rest, its healing system is activated, and this restores the body to a fit state. Even the heart must rest for a moment while it is being recharged for the next contraction, and if there is an interference with this minimum recuperation time, the heart will begin to fail.

We, human beings, as the most complicated of all living systems, must take special care to stop our outer activity, so that internal servicing can be started. This restorative work consists of life support:

Healing; repair and maintenance work.

Defence against invasion, and resistance against illness.

After time out for rest, the organism, refreshed and restored, gets going again. How much time is needed for effective rest?

Watch cats and dogs: they sleep from dusk to dawn, instructed by the going and coming of sunlight, and even then spend half the waking day dozing. They seem to need all that time for efficient internal servicing, and while they are resting, it seems unlikely that their mind has regrets about yesterday or fears of tomorrow.

Young children have the same natural habit: they sleep from seven till seven, and have their morning and afternoon sleep as well. As the saying goes, when they sleep they look like little angels, and sleep like lambs, meaning that they have no worries about yesterday and tomorrow. Theirs is a stress-free sleep. During the period of activity in between these rest periods they brim over with energy, while their tired mother, being the regulating system of the family, tries to keep up with them.

That is how young children get their internal servicing done. And us weary human adults? We are active all day, and when it is dark, we switch on the lights to continue our activity. We have become so obsessed with activity that, even when we are resting, our minds remain busy. Worse, we can no longer stop this mind, because we have no control over it. We learned, at home and at school, to think, but we were never taught to stop thinking, so that even when our body is at rest, our mind is restlessly and uneasily busy, looking for something to do.

And how fit are we as a result of all that activity? Let us answer this question with another: how often do we feel tired, sick, depressed, anxious, and angry, and how many drugs do we adult humans buy and take, to compensate for the lack of fitness? Perhaps the most common use for the over-the-counter drugs such as aspirin and paracetamol is the easing of an abnormal tension, which is stress.

Our Western culture works on the principle of over-loading; you must do your best plus a little bit more. And it is this little extra that causes your regulating system to break down.

Resting is not a luxury. Good quality rest in a stress-free zone is recuperation time, precious time for essential servicing, for defence and for healing.

Life is ongoing and spontaneous activity, it is a creative urge. The self-movement of mobile organisms is an expression of this ceaseless impulse and is experienced as fitness. We need a certain working tension to feel fit, ready for interaction, and it is our natural condition that we must periodically alternate with rest for recuperation.

Sometimes the ongoing activity is temporarily disturbed by an interference from somewhere, but it will soon right itself if this disturbance is not too severe. How does it right itself? It has a regulating system that must keep it balanced while it keeps going.

Imagine a runner: she maintains a dynamic balance that makes her lean forward while she runs, a running balance that keeps her fit and moving. She may sometimes stumble, but she does not fall easily, because she has effective righting systems that put her back in the right balance.

Living means that we run leaning forward in dynamic balance into the immediate future, with powerful righting systems to keep us fit and going. An example of an efficient righting system can be seen during the fall of a cat. The cat always manages to land on its feet, and does it by righting itself accordingly during the fall.

If we catch an illness, we may be sick for a while: we stumble but we normally recover from this, and get back into a state of fitness in well-being. If we don't get better, we go to the doctor and ask why not. We take it for granted, and rightly so, that we should recover, and this belief expresses our deep faith in mother nature as our righting system: she who keeps us balanced and going.

If the weather gets hot, we cool off, and if we are cold, we shiver and warm up; if we feel tired, we rest or sleep. This regulating system that we call mother nature, and that we may call our biological computer, if we want to be more modern, is known by the older medical profession as the *vis medicatrix naturae*. This is the healing force of nature: it is present and working in individual organisms as self-regulation.

Many medical people have become so preoccupied with the

modern artificial techniques of treatment, that they seem to undervalue or even forget the power of this natural healing system. There is always danger in over-riding this natural healing system by an excessive faith in the application of artificial methods of treatment. It is safer to work with it, than to ignore it.

The *vis medicatrix naturae* is a natural biological function of self-regulation: of self-servicing, which is as basic as that biological function for self-moving. We must move to live, but living activity cannot continue without periodic servicing (repair and maintenance), so that our action system must work hand in glove with our internal servicing system.

The action system, which is the system for self-movement, is switched on the moment we get going. While we remain active, our recovery system is turned off, for much the same reason that mechanics cannot service your car while you are driving it. Driving and servicing are not compatible functions because they may get in each other's way.

In the older days of anatomy-based physiology, the action and recovery systems were given the names of the sympathetic and parasympathetic systems respectively, but this division does not convey an accurate picture of the work that is done. W. R. Hess, a Swiss physiologist, pointed out that it is better to look first at the work that is being done, rather than at the anatomical structures.

He named this action system the *ergotropic* system, and the healing system became the *trophotropic* system. The first is an energy-spending system, and the second a recovery (healing) system. There is no need to remember these names, because the names action system and healing (or recovery) system speak for themselves.

When our action system is switched on, we normally have a sense of fitness, that is a proper working tension that makes us feel fit and ready for action. When our recovery system is activated, and the action system is switched off so that we are at rest; we don't feel fit, we feel at ease instead (if this rest is of good quality).

We are only relatively at ease while we are merely resting and therefore not yet relaxed, because we are now still primed for action. If our mind remains busy throughout this resting period, we may get no more than a 'grease and oil change' out of it. The body is resting, but is still ready to jump into action if the mind is still active and thinking about many problems. This organism is not yet relaxing.

Such uneasy ceasing of activity will give a poor quality rest, and does not provide us with a major service.

To reward ourselves with a good quality rest, we must learn to relax, so that we may undergo a major internal service. How does this state of relaxation relate to rest? Relaxation is total rest, it is the ideal resting state, it is resting taken to its utmost limits. Both mind and body are then properly at rest, which means totally at ease.

We may get an idea of the difference between average rest and relaxation from the following facts: at rest, our breathing rate is usually eighteen to twenty respirations per minute, while our pulse rate is about seventy-eight beats in every minute. In relaxation, these values usually drop to under ten (usually four to six) for the breathing rate, and to about sixty for the pulse rate. Such a considerable drop tells us that our metabolic rate is reduced much more in relaxation than at rest.

While we are in a proper resting (relaxed) state, we heal by default, because our healing system is the only system that is now switched on and active; we heal spontaneously.

Rest, in its natural state (such as we see in animals that cannot think all the time like we do), and healing, are linked, so that one cannot occur without the other. If an animal is sick or hurt, it will search naturally (by practical instinct) for a warm, dark and quiet, place. This is a shelter from the world of action, in which it may nurse itself back to health. This means that this dumb animal devotes itself patiently to healing.

Oh, we can't possibly rest, we always say, we have to work, we have a lot to do, a lot of people depend on us, we can't take time off for ourselves, for healing. Or perhaps only grudgingly, so that we work against mother nature, rather than for her and, at the same time, for ourselves. We seem to have become so trapped by our busy life-style that there is no time left for sickness and no place for healing in it.

As a general practitioner, it has always struck me that there is no real room for being ill in this profit-driven culture. People have been made to feel guilty in taking time off from work, as if it were a criminal act to stay home to recover from an illness. Or they may feel threatened by it: 'The boss doesn't like me taking time off, doctor.'

We have become action-addicts, so that we don't even know how to stop and feel comfortable in doing nothing for a while. Yet, we make sure that our car has a regular service: imagine that breaking down. We take better care of our car than of our own body.

Regulation means the following in practice:

(a) We adapt to the outside world. Our body must adapt itself to the shape of the chair when we sit down. When we walk, our body will adapt itself to the shape of the ground. If we are uncomfortable, we change to find a more comfortable position.

We may also change the outer world to suit us and our rational mind can obviously help us to invent ways of reducing noise, cold, and heat, for greater comfort. When someone sneezes, we move away to avoid infection.

Our adaptation to the world around us is achieved through our emotional mind, and this ability to change requires a degree of flexibility of this mind. The emotional mind makes use of the action system for its interaction at the front line with the outside world.

(b) We adapt to our inner world. We have an internal system for inner adjustment which gets its orders from our emotional mind that interacts with the outside world. This internal adapting system (also officially known as our homeostatic system) helps to maintain such interaction, and it keeps us balanced, which means that it makes us fit for interaction, and resistant to illness. We now feel fit for work and also for healing, and for defence against illness, whenever this is needed.

We must understand that this internal system for defence and healing is locked into our interaction in the following way. The organism must take active part in its own healing. Animals do this purely by instinct, like the shelter-seeking dog that we described earlier.

This instinctive programme for self-protection will break down if animals are caged, trapped in a situation that offers no escape. They can no longer do anything useful for themselves in this situation, and it is this inability to help themselves, that makes them lose their biological hope for free living, so that they become apathetic.

Free living is the opportunity to exercise the organism in its practical (effective and appropriate) activity. Living beings have been designed, and built, for action. They are born to act, so that they have a vital need to be practical, to cope with most situations. If this vital need to cope is frustrated, then life itself is frustrated and endangered.

When animals die in captivity, it is death by entrapment, caused by the loss of hope of free living. Such animals suffer from the demoralisation syndrome.

When does our own powerful internal system of resistance (to disorder) and healing break down? When we are trapped. This means that we must get ourselves out of the trap before we can defend ourselves and heal properly. This is why we cannot, and should not, remain passive, when we find we are trapped with cancer.

Let us illustrate the need for rest by looking at what happens to the heart when we reduce its natural rest periods. A heart must rest after every contraction. In this rest period it is being primed for the next contraction. Living organisms do the same.

What happens to the heart if we continue to shorten its rest periods? There comes a time when the rest period becomes less than its minimum, and its priming is disturbed. The heart begins to become disorganised in its work. Because it is now no longer fit for its next contraction, it begins to fail in its task of pumping blood through the body. We call this heart failure. The same failure will occur if the heart must work constantly against an overload. Its resting time becomes inadequate, and normal priming is lost; the heart will eventually fail.

This may also happen with our entire organism. Working on the principle of overload, the current cultural fashion, will lead to organismic failure. This is stress, or coping failure. The middle age burn-out syndrome is a typical example of an organism that has finally gone beyond its coping limits.

It may express itself in an emotional breakdown ('I can't go on, help me') or an organ-system breakdown ('I've got chest pains, help me'). This 'help me' expresses the typical sense of helplessness that we experience in stress. We may know what to do, but we can't bring ourselves to do it.

The overload is, in our culture, rarely a physical overload, but almost always an emotional one. Hard physical work leads only to a pleasant tiredness, but emotional overloading produces fatigue, weariness, exhaustion.

This is not tiredness, but an abnormal emotion of irritable weariness, that should warn us that emotional coping failure is near. It should tell us that we are becoming caught up in a situation with which we cannot cope. We become stressed, we are moving into a trap.

If we get ourselves into such a trap, we have somehow strayed from the normal path of life, in which we are guided by highly practical emotions. We are off the track, like a train that has derailed. We derail into disorder whenever we become trapped, and we must do everything possible to get back on track. And this is a job that we can never leave to others, we must look after it ourselves.

No patient should come to the doctor without saying (if not to the doctor, at least to herself: what can I do to help myself?) This attitude is so important for any kind of healing, that we may say no proper healing is possible without it. The patient who comes to some therapist with the attitude of: 'Here I am, poor helpless me, please heal me', may have to wait a long time for healing, if it happens at all.

The late Professor J. H. Schultz, one of the greatest psychotherapists in Europe, created his now famous system of autogenic training to give people the means to take an active part in their own healing, whatever the nature of the illness. Autogenic means self-generated.

TAKING AN ACTIVE ATTITUDE

If ever the saying: 'To do a job properly, do it yourself' is true, it is here. Your job is first and foremost to get out of the bad emotional trap of believing that you must die from cancer. This will be the topic of the third part of the book that we shall introduce here.

By all means get all the help you can in your effort to open up this trap, and escape from it. We shall come back to this, and it is enough for now to realise how important this is.

First: you don't have to die from cancer. This 'I must die' notion is a bad myth that can be a hazard to your recovery, if you believe in it.

Second: you can't heal properly in any kind of entrapment, and especially not in this kind of entrapment with a wrong belief. You can only work against healing if you stay in it.

By taking an active role in your own healing, by getting into the driver's seat yourself and taking stock of your situation, you can escape any kind of trap and begin to work towards your own healing. Don't be a passive patient. That does not work.

Once you have taken charge, you may now delegate some jobs to others, to doctors who become your assistants, for example. But you must do this from a position of strength, so that you are no longer a passive, helpless patient. You should throw off the paralysing passivity that allows you to slide further into despair. How this can be done will be discussed later.

We can be trapped physically, but we may also fall into an emotional trap, and we shall see that such an emotional trap is often far more serious. We know from the study of the survivors of concentration camps and prisoner-of-war camps, and from experience with peace-time emotional traps.

Very important work has been done in this field by Professor Jan Bastiaans of the Netherlands. It is significant that he has also worked with cancer patients. Many cancer patients, he found, are emotionally locked-in, and incapable of freedom of emotional expression. They urgently need to be liberated from this emotional captivity.

People who die a psychogenic death, said Professor Jores, die in the gaol of their own ego, they die in their hopelessness. He quotes Plügge, another researcher, speaking of hope as a fundamental anthropological fact (pages 111, 122–7). He is saying that hope is an indispensable factor in the existence of human beings, that it is part of being alive.

These peacetime emotional traps are emotional concentration camps that can be harmful, as many soldiers and concentration camp survivors found out even after the wars. With a return to peace-time living, for example, angina and diabetes, and other pre-war problems, returned.

Distress of the emotional mind in entrapment, in finding itself in a situation with which it cannot cope, is what the term stress really means. Stress is often defined as a load, but this is a definition that comes from physical science. Stress is an overload, and this means that we are not coping with the situation.

And when is something an emotional overload? Whenever we feel trapped by it, when we feel helpless and hopeless, whenever we cannot cope and give up trying to cope. A difficult situation is not yet a trap, because there is always hope for a solution and a door open somewhere, an escape route for the emotional mind. We can still cope with a difficult situation, but we can no longer cope in a trap, because all our efforts are in vain. A trap is a closed situation, and there is no escape possible.

It does not matter whether our rational mind recognises this situation as a trap. As long as our emotional mind views the situation as a trap, it is a trap for the organism.

Our emotional mind guides our behaviour, and also regulates the internal functions to support it. Normal emotions are therefore our practical guides to behaviour. Practical means appropriate; purposeful and effective in most situations of living and surviving.

This also means that wrong emotions, if they are present too long or too intensely, guide us into trouble. They disorganise us in our behaviour and in our internal workings, because they misguide us. They are no longer practical, no longer compatible with health. Such wrong emotions are inappropriate emotions for normal living, they are abnormal.

Part Three

THE PSYCHOLOGY
OF CANCER

Chapter Nine

THE NORMAL ORGANISM

Our emotional mind is involved in practically everything that the body does, because this emotional mind has the important task of instructing the body in all its activities. Our daily routine activities, which vary little from day to day, may be carried out more or less automatically by the body, but more changeable activities depend on the emotional mind for direct instructions. Anything that the body does, it can only do under instruction from the emotional mind.

Our organism may be compared to a company in which the director is our emotional mind and the workers our body. The emotional mind organises the body for its various activities. The experience of fear, for example, is the practical organisation of our body for flight. If we were resting before that, then our body is reorganised from its activity of recuperation to that of fight or flight. The body is always engaged in some kind of programme; one of activity or of recovery. A body does nothing on its own, it is guided by sensory (instinctual) or emotional directives.

This emotional mind directs by feelings that we may or may not be aware of. Our awareness, or lack of it, is not relevant to the work of the emotional mind. Feelings are instructions for the body, after all, not information for the rational knowing mind. From a practical point of view, we don't need to know anything about our feelings.

Every feeling (emotion or sensation) is a complete message. A feeling is a complicated instruction for the body, no matter how fleeting it may seem, and how little we may know about its existence. Every normal feeling and memory is part and parcel of an action programme.

If we want to know a feeling or memory, we have to lift it out of

101

its programme, and examine it as a separate fact, so that we usually lose sight of the fact that it exists for action, that it is part of an action programme. It is like taking a word out of a story, and looking at it by itself: we have lost the story that goes with it, because we are seeing it out of context.

If we wish to better understand this emotional mind, we must first understand what the body is for. We need to understand how this emotional mind works, because it plays a central role in the problem of psychological cancer.

OUR BODY EXISTS FOR THE PURPOSE OF ACTION

The body is built for continuous action, for being busy with the business of living. We only need to look around us; ants, bees, cats, dogs, and humans are always on the go during their waking hours. Even bacteria have means of getting around. Our body is a practical means for moving around.

Higher animals require time for resting from their intense activities; they need to stop being busy at regular periods to recuperate from action, and to get ready for more activity. This is time for essential repair and maintenance work.

Why our body and mind have been designed and built for action, and why we exist for the sake of action, is not our concern here.

Being active does not mean that we indulge in random activity. Living action is always directed activity, action that is motivated. Motivated behaviour means behaviour brought about by some emotion. It is behaviour that has been instructed to proceed in a practical way by some feeling.

Biologically speaking, our task in life is to survive, and we have emotions to instruct and guide the body in its survival activities. We learn from past experience; our emotional mind can distil practical memories out of this experience, memories that can be usefully incorporated into future action.

In lower organisms, the directions for activity are wired into the body as instincts; such instincts are primitive and fairly rigid instructions for living that are built into the nervous system. Learning here involves rewiring the system, which is not all that easy.

Emotions are different from instincts only in that they are more flexible and advanced instructions that can better adapt themselves to changing situations. We have many more emotions than we have instincts because, as human beings, we are more flexible, and we can adapt better to changes in any situation that we are in. This makes emotions more practical guides to survival. Learning is now easier because it does not require rewiring, only reprogramming.

Instincts are usually experienced as urgent sensations which cannot be put off, at least, not for very long. We have an instinct to breathe, for example, and this is an instruction that will not allow us to put off breathing for long, because it is a very strong need.

Sensations and emotions are instructions for the body. They are feelings that guide the body in all its activities. Instincts are instructions that are always the same; they never vary, while feelings are changeable.

Without instructions, a washing machine does nothing; without instructions, a computer does nothing; without instructions, a living body does nothing. Washing machines have a knob with different settings, and these are instructions for washing. The settings form the 'washing mind'. Washing, as a function, means more than a machine that does the washing motions; washing makes use of this machine to do the job. Without its instruction, the machine is not a washing machine. The task of washing can be performed by different means, by hand, for example, so that the machine is only one possible way of doing the job. The task (function) belongs to the mind, while the unchanging routine of execution belongs to the body.

Computers have software that consists of a set of instructions for computing. The software is the 'computing mind' that makes use of the computer equipment to perform the task of computing.

Living beings have a mind that is also a set of instructions for living. This mind may be a primitive instinctive mind, but all higher organisms have a more advanced emotional mind.

The emotional mind stirs the body into action, and we may even say that the emotional mind makes use of the body to achieve its task of keeping the organism alive. A still, motionless body does not have an emotional mind to run it, because such a body is not doing anything, and it needs no emotions to direct it. This is why we feel emotionally neutral in relaxation; the emotional mind has switched off because it is not needed.

Our rational mind can become active while the emotional mind is at ease, calm and detached, and in neutral gear.

When we see someone in action, what we actually see is the emotional mind in action. This emotional mind makes the body do whatever needs to be done, so that it makes use of the body to fulfil its practical purpose of living. This is why we say that the mind is not in the body, but the body is in the mind.

The mind is the flexible and changeable part of our organism, while the body is the fixed routine aspect of the organism.

We may also express it in this way; the body is the child of the emotional mind, not its parent. The mind is the parent of the body, and not the other way around. And when the body does something wrong, we look to its parent, the emotional mind, to ask why the child received the wrong instruction.

When something goes wrong with the functions of the body, and we focus here on defence and healing, we should also look to the emotional mind and ask what went wrong with normal defence and healing. When we catch a cold, we must also ask why we got it, rather than only wonder how the virus managed to enter our system.

Little children and higher animals such as cats and dogs have only an emotional mind to guide them in their activities. Adult human beings also have a second mind, a rational mind, to assist the emotional mind, but this rational mind can only advise the emotional mind. The rational mind cannot take over this job of instructing the body as to what proper action is to be taken, because the emotional mind sits at the controls.

This emotional mind may, or may not, take any notice of this advice, sound and logical as it may be according to rational logic. The emotional mind has its own emotional logic on which it operates. That may not be compatible with any rational advice, so that this rational advice will be ignored.

The emotional mind is in the driver's seat. The rational mind is limited to staying in the passenger's seat, from where it can only give advice to the driver.

The emotional mind, sitting in the driver's seat, is responsible for anything that happens in (and with) the body, either by direct or indirect instruction. If anything goes wrong, we must always look at the emotional mind, in case this was no accident in the body, but the result of a wrong emotional instruction.

In this book we are not concerned with behaviour, but with the internal self-servicing system that is responsible for defence against any disturbance. We are also concerned with healing, with damage repair. And we focus on defence against our self-infection with cancer cells, and on healing from it.

If something has gone wrong with this function of defence or healing, we must ask if this is due to some internal material accident, or to a wrong emotional instruction.

If we trace these wrong emotional instructions back to their origin, we shall find that they were born in stress. We know that stress interferes with defence and healing. We become sick more severely and more easily, and recovery takes longer. Stress by itself already disorganises defence and healing, but wrong emotional instructions, born in stress, can do extra harm by misdirecting the body towards self-destruction.

We may even say that it is precisely this disorganisation that makes a misdirection possible; causing initial disorder prior to moving in a different direction is a recognised and effective political strategy. The initial disorder allows the system to shake loose from its previous path. Misdirection is born in the disorder created by stress.

A normal emotional mindset promotes good defence and healing because that is part of practical survival. A wrong emotional mindset in stress has a disorganising effect on healing and defence. But, worse: a wrong instruction can actively work against defence and healing, and may work against survival.

For those who are interested, let me try to make clear what tension is, because the difference between normal tension and stress is not generally known.

Action, and movement in general, requires tension. Now, to be able to act, to do useful work in keeping ourselves going, we need a sufficient degree of working tension. Without this, we would not feel fit. When we are relaxed, that strange lazy feeling of: 'I am so comfortable that I don't feel like stirring', tells us that our muscles are limp and off-duty.

In this relaxed state we are underpowered, and do not feel fit, yet we have a great sense of ease and well-being. We may experience an inability to get going in depression, and even in boredom, but this is associated with a negative feeling, a paralysed feeling that is anything but a sense of comfort and ease.

To become fit from this state of ease, we have to do whatever we usually do, when we wake up from a good quality sleep in order to get going again: we have to call our muscles back to work, and we yawn and stretch and pump the muscles a bit. This produces the needed working tension, so that we feel fit and ready to go. We mobilise our organism for action. The so-called *antigravity muscles* contract and produce that typical sensation of lightness that we take for granted as we act; it allows us to move the body.

Watch top tennis players give a little shuffle now and then to stay fit and flexible and primed to the optimal degree of working tension.

When we have a *normal working tension*, we feel fit and ready for any action, for play or work. Things that we have to do are a challenge that we take for granted: *we are coping fit.* We have a feeling of fitness-in-well-being.

When we are relaxed, we have, instead, a great sense of ease-in-well-being, but we don't feel fit. We actually feel much too comfortable to bother about moving and getting going, and this feeling is due to the utter limpness of our muscle system.

When we are stressed, we have neither a sense of fitness nor a sense of ease. We feel unfit, we feel nervous and irritable, and weary. We have no sense of well-being, but feel unwell and uneasy instead. We feel unfit and abnormally tense in our body and in our emotional mind. Our muscle system is neither limp, nor geared efficiently to action. It is disorganised and often in a state of useless spasm, with an abnormal quality of tension.

Stress begins when our normal working tension goes overboard, past its normal limits, when we are too tense to be effective. This abnormal and excessive tension works like a brake on our efficiency.

Chapter Ten

THE EMOTIONAL MIND EXISTS TO GUIDE THE BODY IN ACTION

Emotions guide our organism in most of its day-to-day contacts with the world, and they play an essential part in the maintenance of our well-being. They are important in producing and maintaining our state of well-being (that is when we say: I am well), and our feeling of well-being (when we say: I feel well).

Wrong (negative) emotions are harmful when they are too strong and too long: they are abnormal in quality and toxic to our system.

Human life is far more complicated than that of animals, because human beings have a capacity for abstract thinking, and because our emotional capacity is greater. We can experience a greater variety of emotions than animals can, and these are typically the emotions that make us human in the best sense of the word. But, equally, those emotions can lead us into distressing difficulties and traps.

An example of the first kind is compassion. We may well say that this is the highest human emotion. An example of the other kind is guilt, and we may also say, with good reason, that guilt is the most useless and poisonous emotion we humans are capable of.

Guilt is an abnormal emotion, because it reveals a state of disorganisation of the emotional mind. We must not confuse guilt with a sense of responsibility which stands on the same level with compassion. Guilt is a disordered sense of responsibility, an impractical and harmful stress-emotion.

To understand what happens to the emotional mind in distress, we must first understand the meaning of frustration which is the main sign of the emotional mind in trouble. Frustration is our original negative feeling, it is the first feeling-sensation of distress that the newborn baby is capable of experiencing. The organism in trouble experiences a basic and primitive feeling of undifferentiated frustration. We could say that frustration is the mother of all negative feelings, meaning that all individual negative feelings have later grown out of it. Frustration remains as the background feeling in all negative emotions, such as anger, hate, hostility, envy, jealousy, and the anxious forms of negative emotions: anxiety, panic, self-doubt, guilt, shame, inferiority, and so on.

Anger and anxiety, for example, are abnormal (and therefore useless) feelings. They may seem to be very different feelings in the adult, but they have the same origin in childhood: they are both born out of the source feeling of frustration.

A baby's first distress is a general frustration, and that is why it can be so difficult to make out, at least in the early weeks, whether it is angry, hungry, in pain or simply wet.

Feelings guide our behaviour, and feeling is a general term for all sensations and emotions. We have sensations such as thirst, hunger, sleepiness, and the urge to go to the toilet. Sensations are guides to our basic body care, as it were, and we experience their guiding action as a need to act appropriately.

Sensations are guiding feelings that are usually quite clearly localised in some part of the body: air-hunger in the chest, food-hunger in the stomach region, a full bladder in the lower abdomen, thirst in the mouth, and so on. The word sensation describes our experience of these feelings, and if we wish to refer to their motive (driving) power, we call them instincts.

Emotions, being higher feelings, and therefore more flexible, are more general feelings, because they have lost this direct connection with a specific part of our body.

We can see this arrangement with all our higher functions; the higher they are, the less clearly they are localised in one or other part of the body or brain. If we think of emotions as general sensations, then we can understand that the emotional mind is as much part of the organism as digestion is. The only difference is that the mind is not so clearly localised in our organism: we cannot point to its place in it.

Emotions continuously guide our interaction with the world around us, and the guiding emotions do this in various ways. Primitive emotions are very strong, and they simply force us to do what mother nature thinks we should, so that we, as the conscious personality, have no choice but to obey such instructions. These primitive emotions are often difficult to distinguish from instincts (sensations).

Less primitive emotions don't push so strongly; they only urge us to do certain things. The least primitive emotions, which are the most sophisticated ones, no longer push for action, or at least, not so insistently. We may delay the activity that they insist on, if this is more to our practical benefit.

Examples of sensations that are irresistible are: air-hunger (the need or urge to breathe), sleepiness (the need to sleep), thirst (the need to drink), and itch (the need to scratch). I have added the almost unnecessary descriptions of the quality of the sensations in parentheses, to draw attention to the fact that these urges (needs) that we experience as sensations are clearly instructions for action: sleeping, drinking, scratching, and so on, are all practical activities.

Examples of powerful primitive emotions are: love, parental feelings, sexual needs, rage, fury and fear. Such feelings are so close to strong sensations that we often cannot tell the difference. Primitive sensations may also be called instincts, if we look at the behaviour that is the result of their urgent pushing. Our powerfully primitive emotions work much like instincts.

Examples of sophisticated (higher) emotions are: mature love, compassion, responsibility, and the feeling for beauty, moral, religious, ethical, and other such emotions. Generally, these are contemplative feelings. They allow us look at, or listen to, some situation without needing to operate on it: a painting, a landscape, a concert. There is no longer any urge to go into immediate action, and to manipulate the situation. We may fold our arms and remain quite motionless while looking or listening with great patience. This is an achievement of a higher order, and only a mature adult has this ability; little children and animals are still influenced strongly by a biological impatience, an urge to action. They cannot remain still long enough.

Our normal feelings are practical guides to our behaviour; the more primitive the feeling is, the more primitive the activity that it pushes us into doing. Primitive emotions are strong (intense), and push us with great driving power into primitive acts. Aggression impels us to attack, while fear forces us to run from danger.

These primitive feelings are our original jungle feelings that are geared to our immediate survival, and that is why we call them practical. They are strong, effective and purposeful in keeping us alive here and now.

We have many more practical emotions than we have been able to recognise and label. Most of these do their work silently and quickly, gone before we can know them. Cross a busy road, for example, and what is it that leads you safely across? Feelings that you are not even aware of, except perhaps for a sense of caution. We don't know that it is safe to cross, we only feel it. We experience it as a gut-feeling rather than as explicit knowledge.

This is an important point. Feelings are not there for us to know, they don't need to become conscious knowledge, they only have to push us in the right direction. When we talk about the unconscious mind or the subconscious mind, we really mean the emotional mind.

Feelings are not created to inform the rational mind about the world, they are produced to push our organism into immediate action, and that is practical. We don't have to stop to think, because we don't have the time. We jump into action. We jump at something to attack it, or we jump away from it to escape it. The sudden appearance of a snake in the garden will make us jump away. The mere sight of the snake compels us to jump; we don't need to stop to think rationally about the situation, because that could be fatal.

In jungle conditions we have no time to say: 'Hmm, let me see now: is this animal that looks like a tiger, dangerous for me? Is that snake a poisonous one? And what reason would I have to run away from it?' We would be eaten up or fatally bitten long before we could finish this train of thought.

Useful points to remember about feelings are therefore:

Feelings are practical, but only for as long as they have a normal intensity, and that means as long as they are not too long and not too strong. Too long and too strong means abnormal in quality.

For practical living, such feelings have to be just right; they must not make us feel too little and not too much. Too cold is harmful, too hot is equally harmful.

Too strong emotions make us drunk, they intoxicate us, so that we are no longer in control of ourselves. They disorganise us: they push us over the limit of practical regulation, so that they send us over the edge of our practical limits of coping. If emotions are not strong enough, they underpower us, so that we cannot get going.

Feelings have practical limits: they have a minimum strength (threshold) and a maximum strength (ceiling). If they are under the threshold or above the ceiling, they are no longer useful, because their strength is either not enough or too much. But this also means that they are abnormal in their guiding quality. They are now no longer reliable guides to action, and we can no longer trust them to tell us the practical truth about reality. In addition to this, they may even be harmful to us. In anger, panic or depression, we have distorted (exaggerated) notions about our reality, abnormal ideas that are born out of such wrong emotions. Later, when we have recovered from them, we may realise how inappropriate and impractical they were.

All feelings change in their guiding quality when they change in intensity. Being merely annoyed implies a different kind of action to be taken (if any) from the attack-urging feeling of rage, for example.

Abnormal emotions are practical emotions that have become too strong, so intense that they disorganise our system. Whatever else we may say about them, they are impractical and useless. Their presence should warn us that we are not coping with the current situation. This situation has become too much for us to cope, we are not in control of it, and all these abnormal emotions express this fact of not coping. We are frustrated in our attempt to cope. We have failed in this situation.

That is why frustration is the mother of all abnormal emotions and why all these abnormal emotions are variations of the same primitive feeling of frustration. Not coping is failure, and this is the frustration of an organism that is born to cope.

Anger, anxiety, depression, hate, hostility, envy, jealousy: don't they all spell out frustration? When do we feel these emotions? When we can't do anything about the situation, when we have a sense of failure, of not coping. That means when we are stuck with a situation that we cannot do anything about. That situation is a trap.

The second point to remember about our emotions is that we don't have to be conscious of them in the sense of knowing anything about them; we are only just as much conscious of them as we need to be, to act on them. We need to be aware of our feelings only enough for them to do their work, which is to move us into action.

The third point to remember about feelings is that they are by nature practical, which means useful for surviving. These are the feelings that we call normal. We usually don't pay any special attention to these feelings while we are being silently and efficiently guided by them. Such extra attention would only interfere with an efficient performance.

Abnormal means inappropriate and, therefore, no longer useful for us in staying alive and well. These are no longer of any practical use to us, so that they can now only mis-guide us in our interactions. We do and say things in anger that we would not do or say if we were calm and sober.

Emotions work on us like alcohol: a little wine is good for the heart, but too much intoxicates us. The same can be said of emotion. We become drunk and useless with too much of it. It intoxicates our brain. Too much means abnormal, and abnormal means disorganising. Too much and too long of emotions and alcohol will damage our system. When we are very angry, we behave like drunks. We are a danger on the road because we have lost our normal control.

Our normal emotions organise us for effective and appropriate living, for our outer practical behaviour, and efficient inner regulation (healing and resistance).

Abnormal emotions dis-organise our system. They are no longer proper guides for the maintenance of life with its internal regulations and adjustments. They are entirely false messages for healing and defence against illness.

We experience abnormal sensations and emotions in distressing situations, and all these negative emotions are variations of one single primitive and disabling emotion: frustration. In the next chapters we shall examine this important parent of all negative feeling in greater detail.

Chapter Eleven

THE DISTRESSED ORGANISM

A situation becomes distressing when we can no longer cope with it. The distress is not limited to an upset of the mind, but soaks through the entire normal organism, just as adding vinegar to coffee spoils the entire contents of the cup.

We are born to cope. We have been biologically designed and built to cope; to live and to keep living our everyday life. Coping refers to the practical management of our everyday living, and implies that we are capable of dealing actively and effectively with almost any situation that might come up; and that we derive some practical benefit from it. We get food, water, and other living necessities, from the situation.

If we can no longer cope with a life situation, it means that we have lost control, that we are not managing it any more; we no longer get any practical benefit from it, and it might even harm us.

There is a difference between a difficult situation with which we cope, even if we are struggling, and a situation with which we are no longer coping.

If the situation is difficult, we may still feel that we have control over it, and that we are managing it well enough, so that we feel challenged to try to continue to cope with it.

When the situation becomes so complicated, that we are no longer managing it adequately, it means we are failing to cope with it. We can no longer experience this situation as a challenge to get something positive out of it. We can now only experience this scene as a threat to our security and well-being. Instead of expecting any advantage from it, we fear that it may harm us.

A situation like this is no longer just difficult, it is now an impossible situation, a situation beyond our coping capacity. It is a distressing situation and what we experience in it is distress (stress). The accompanying feeling is one of frustration.

Stress means coping failure. It is a failure of practical management of the current situation. Practical management is being able to cope normally; our management skills are mostly effective and useful.

Our coping capacity is limited. We cannot cope with extreme situations and events in the outside world. Natural disasters are crises situations that grow beyond the capacity of our practical emotional mind for everyday management. We have limits to our normal human dimension of experience, and we may become aware of these, when we meet a situation that is outsize, too large, too deep, too high, too painful, too much for our practical coping size.

If we stand at the very edge of a deep cliff, for example, we become uncomfortably aware of our practical limitations. We can't cope with that enormous drop and we become disorientated and dizzy. We are now no longer in familiar territory for our practical human size. We are confronted with a shocking view that is outside our familiar human dimension of experience and beyond our practical coping capacity. We lose confidence in our ability to remain balanced, and become afraid that we might topple over. We experience the threat of a coping failure, of stress.

There are also extreme situations that can affect the personal part of our emotional mind, so that we are personally and individually in trouble. Our personality (as the personalised region of our emotional mind) also has its limits of practical coping and will be disorganised and impractical outside these boundaries.

Now, being out of our personal depth and in a disorganised state, we are liable to make wrong personal decisions we may later regret.

A failure situation is a situation in which we no longer feel fit to cope. Instead, we experience frustration. Feeling frustrated means feeling angry, anxious (frightened, nervous), useless, and helpless. We feel that we are now no longer in control of the situation, that we can do nothing useful about it, that we are no longer fit to manage it. We then feel helpless, weary, and irritable.

Frustration is the demoralising experience of finding ourselves in a situation in which we can no longer act usefully. We are frustrated in our need to cope actively with a situation, and because we are self-aware as human beings, we also become conscious of our helpless frustration.

It is important to understand why I keep making this frequent reference to action. We are born to act, to cope, to manage, to be active in any situation, except when we decide to relax. Our biological being demands that we do something useful about any situation that we are in. It is a deep-seated instinct that must be satisfied if we wish to continue living.

We must do something useful, and if we find that we cannot manage this, we feel trapped; helpless, hopeless, demoralised.

During distress, our entire biological system is disorganised, and our emotional mind is unfit for coping. There is no practical difference between having stomach pains (a sign of our disorganised body) and having a poor self-image (a sign of our disorganised emotional mind). Both symptoms are merely signs of disorganisation in our system that is designed to act without such handicaps. And it is in a stressed organism, that all kinds of infections can take hold and flourish.

During stress our emotions are no longer practical and reliable instructions for living a normal life. Emotions that we experience during stress may fool us into thinking that reality is how we feel about it. When we wake up in the middle of the night in panic, we may feel that the world is one big dark threat, that life is too awful to continue. Once the attack is over and we feel better, we wonder how we could have thought the world was such a bad place.

Panic makes us believe in woe and disaster because we make the mistake of not realising that the disorganised emotion of high anxiety is no longer a reliable guide to reality. Don't believe in what your emotional mind tells you when you are anxious or angry. This emotional mind is in disarray and not working properly, no longer a reliable and practical guide to reality. The medical term for loss of normal function is dysfunction. The disorganised mind is a dysfunctional mind.

Stress is an emotional load that is too heavy to carry, an abnormal load, a weight of abnormal quality.

The heaviest emotional load of all is a death sentence. This may be real or imagined (such as the imagined death sentence with cancer) but, in any case, it is a load that is too heavy to carry for even the strongest mind.

It is entirely beyond the emotional carrying (coping) capacity of most people, so that we sag and crumple under its weight, and give up. We become apathetic, emotionally numbed, and then accept death as inevitable. Even if our rational mind knows better, our emotional mind may still believe in the false death sentence, and continue on the road to unnecessary self-destruction. How can the rational mind teach the emotional mind the truth about this danger?

The rational mind, as we said, has no direct connection with the body computer, and cannot over-ride the emotional mind in the driver's seat. Therefore, we must first switch off the dominating emotional mind if we wish to put the rational mind to work. Strong feelings silence the rational mind. Only an emotional mind that is at rest and at ease, lacking any strong feelings, will be open to reason, willing to listen to advice from the rational mind.

We must first learn to neutralise our emotional mind by relaxing; we must learn to calm it down and to reduce its dominating strength before we can think rationally. The emotional mind activates the body, and we can settle the emotional mind by relaxing the body. We rest the body so that we can be at ease and start thinking.

An emotional mind is always a practical mind for action, while a rational mind is a theoretical mind for thinking at rest. We use relaxation to bring the emotional mind to a state of rest and neutrality, so that it is under control, and open to appropriate suggestions from the rational mind in the form of concrete words or pictures (visual images). It then translates these into corresponding feelings that are passed on to the nervous system as messages for the body. This is what happens in hypnosis, in which the subject's rational mind is replaced by that of the hypnotist. In auto-hypnosis (self-hypnosis), we use our own rational mind to guide the emotional mind, and this is much better, because we can then practise this method independently, and as often as we need to maintain improvement.

Our emotional mind is the software, and our body the hardware of that total system that we call our organism. This organism has to live and go on living, and it has the necessary set of software programs, as well as the needed hardware to put these programs into practice. Our emotional mind gives the instructions, and the body puts them into practice, it enacts these instructions. Our nervous system acts as the middle man between the emotional mind and organ systems. It translates feeling-messages for the body into appropriate code for our organ systems; messages for action and for the necessary support of that activity.

The emotional mind and the body are inseparable parts of the same organism. The body cannot function without its guiding emotions. But we also see that wrong emotions create havoc in this body instead of guiding it in an efficient and practical way of doing things. They mis-guide it, and cause damage to the system.

I repeat that this harmful effect appears only if these wrong emotions are constantly at work. Occasional negative emotions are little hiccups that have no lasting effect on the system.

Wrong emotions are abnormal in two ways: they are no longer practical emotions. They are poor and useless guides for the body; they are potentially harmful as well. They could guide this body in a wrong direction.

An emotional mind that has been corrupted can cause the body to self-destruct. That is why it must be restored to its normal practical order. A wrong emotion is like a computer virus: get rid of it before it damages your normal programs for living!

The wrong belief that you must necessarily die from cancer is such a software virus that it has infected the emotional mind. This book is therefore somewhat like anti-virus software; it shows you how to get rid of the malignant virus in your emotional mind.

THE NORMAL EMOTIONAL MIND

We have emotions for a practical reason: they are necessary guides to normal living. Normal emotions push us into practical action and guide us in certain ways of behaving in the world around us, to our benefit. They tell our body what to do and where or when to do it. The nervous system already contains its own wired-in instructions of how to perform all these activities, and how to support them internally. It only sends appropriate messages to the organs and systems of the body that must carry out these instructions.

The emotional mind decides on what is to be done, and the body (via the nervous system) listens to the instructions and carries them out. The body listens to the emotional mind as the child listens to its parent.

Anything that takes place in the body, any action that has to do with practical living, with life-sustaining behaviour, is determined by the emotional mind. Life-sustaining and life-promoting actions happen only on direct instruction from the emotional mind.

If the emotional mind has been programmed with the wrong software, then our behaviour will also be abnormal because the body will receive wrong emotional messages and carry out these faulty instructions.

Hysterical paralysis of a leg has nothing to do with the leg itself. The patient, as the total organism, can't move her leg. A neurologist checks out the leg and says that there is nothing wrong with it, and he is right. There is nothing wrong with the patient's legs (with the hardware itself), but everything is wrong with the way it has been programmed for moving. The fault lies with the practical use of the leg.

Such a paralysed leg is useless, and if this is due to wrong emotional instructions, then there is a virus in the emotional mind.

This patient cannot use the leg, and everything happens as if the emotional mind is now instructing the body: don't walk. The body carries this out. It performs the act of making sure that no walking will take place. The emotional virus has put a taboo on walking.

This is not far removed from everyday life. The rational mind may advise: 'There is no money in that', but the emotional mind may say: 'do it anyway'. Tell a smoker to stop smoking, and he cannot do it. He is unable to perform the act of not smoking, because the emotional mind says: 'smoke, don't stop.'

The false notion held by the typical cancer patient, that he or she must die from cancer, is a software virus. Unless this virus is eradicated the body will simply carry out the instruction. Even while the rational mind disbelievingly says nonsense, the emotional mind commands: Die!, and will be obeyed.

Mr TCP loses his appetite and other interests, and will feel very helpless because there is nothing he can do to change the sentence. He feels hopeless because he is convinced by now that no one can save him from this dreadful fate. Soon he will lose weight and begin to look awful, and all for nothing.

Mr TCP's emotional mind, ordinarily practical and efficient software, has been infected with a virus.

It is amazing, though, how this typical cancer patient comes alive when this is clearly understood by him. The terminal picture that Mr TCP presents is soon gone, no matter what happens with the biological cancer inside the body at this early stage.

The debilitating side-effects from some forms of chemotherapy or radiotherapy may spoil this picture. But even these side-effects can (with some effort) be incorporated into the right software; if you feel miserable, it may help to think of how the cancer cells will feel, because they are weaker than your normal cells. Cancer cells are not the monstrously strong cells they have been made out to be in the fearful lay public's imagination.

Chapter Twelve

THE NATURE OF ENTRAPMENT

Sometimes we may find ourselves in situations that we cannot do anything about. The reason for this helpless inability may be inside our emotional mind or outside it in the world of things and other people. For one reason or another we are stuck with a situation that is too much for our emotional mind to cope with. We are unhappy with it, yet we can't get away from it.

Let us look more closely at the situation that a typical cancer patient is caught up in so that we may understand the danger better.

We possess a practical emotional mind that is effective in dealing with a variety of situations. Now we find ourselves in a situation that we cannot manage in our usual practical way. We cannot find an adequate solution for the problem, we don't know what to do about it, and it seems as if we are stuck with it. The situation is beyond our coping capacity.

That we cannot solve it is one thing, and we can always keep trying. But sometimes it seems that we cannot get out of it because our emotional mind won't even let us try to escape, or because the complicated situation itself does not allow it. In either case, we cannot escape it.

We cannot stay in such a situation either. It is unbearable for our emotional mind so there is a growing need to escape, if not in a normal way, then in an abnormal way. The situation is intolerable.

This is our problem situation: a predicament that we cannot solve, escape from, nor stay in.

Coping means managing and controlling the situation and, if necessary, changing it to our practical benefit. We always gain something from coping, even if it is only preventing ourselves from being harmed by the problem.

When the situation is beyond coping, when it is too difficult to manage, we experience a loss of the normal sense of fitness and dealing ability that we take for granted. We now have a feeling of powerlessness, a paralysing helplessness that is part of the general frustration, so that the situation may now harm us.

If the situation becomes too difficult to manage, we shall also experience a sense of failure, a coping failure that is announced by the appearance of anxiety. Anxiety is always a sign of distress. It informs us that we are not managing the situation to our benefit, that we may become hurt by it. Anxiety is always helpless anxiety.

Fear, on the other hand, is practical and effective in managing the situation. Look how fast we run for safety. We are like a champion sprinter.

Like anxiety, anger is always a signal of distress, of coping failure. We become angry if we cannot manage the situation to our practical benefit. Anger is always helpless anger, it is the frustration of assertiveness and aggression.

ENTRAPMENT

What kind of situation is this then, in which we find ourselves too helpless and powerless to do anything useful? It is a trap, an entrapment situation. If there is one condition that an organism (built and born to cope) cannot endure, it is entrapment. It makes its life a futile thing, an absurdity. We are organisms that have a biological need to cope.

What use are sense organs if we are prevented from perceiving the world with them? Where is the sense of having muscles if we are not allowed to exercise them? What is the use of being a practical organism that is born to cope and move freely, if it is trapped? What is an organism (that lives to cope just as an eye exists to see) when it is trapped? It is a frustrated being if it cannot do what it is born to do. This frustrated organism becomes depressed and demoralised. We may not be aware of it, but this is why we feel demoralised in entrapment. We feel like a useless eye or leg, we feel like a useless organism feels: helpless, powerless, hopeless. Our existence now seems futile. These are confessions of powerlessness, of helpless impotence: I can't do anything about it; I can't help myself; I must not do or say anything to upset others, even if it is to save myself.

This powerlessness is a paralysis of the practical emotional mind.

What would prevent us from staying in a trap without harm? Why can't we just accept it, and live in it contentedly? We can't do it because entrapment is intolerable. An unbearable feeling forces us to escape in much the same way that severe pain compels our hand to withdraw from a flame, and an irresistible urge makes us breathe again when we try to hold our breath for too long.

If even our inventive rational mind cannot help us to find a normal escape route for our organism, then our disorganised emotional mind will search for an abnormal one, and may find it in illness or death. Whatever happens, we cannot stay unaffected and unharmed by entrapment.

These are the characteristics of an entrapment situation, as we saw earlier in this chapter: The situation is beyond our coping power, meaning that we can do nothing useful to change it, and to help ourselves. We cannot escape from it; a trap is a closed situation. We cannot stay in it either, because of the enormous sense of frustration that urges us to do something about it.

What we experience in this situation is stress. Stress is the experience of finding ourselves in a trap, in a situation that we can't handle, and cannot walk away from, but cannot bear much longer either. It is an impossible situation, and something must give if it continues for too long.

THE STAGES OF ENTRAPMENT

Finding ourselves in a trap, we become angry and anxious, and we struggle to find an escape route, any escape route, if we cannot solve it to our satisfaction. If all this searching is in vain, we come to the painful realisation that there is nothing we can do about it. Now our anger and anxiety will fade and we will cease our struggle; we begin to feel helpless about this hopeless situation: what's the use of trying?

We become demoralised, depressed, resigned, apathetic.

There are roughly three stages of entrapment:

Denial. We experience a shock if the entrapment is sudden and unexpected. There is a sense of unreality about it: 'This can't be happening to me, it's a bad dream, it can't be true'.

Rebellion. We rebel against fate: 'Why should this happen to me, of all people, I don't deserve this, it's not fair'.

Resignation. We lose the sense of rebellion and now resign ourselves to the hard reality of the situation. The frustrated emotional mind becomes depressed as the sense of outrage and rebellion fades. If the situation is not resolved, then this resignation becomes abnormal, and we need help.

Depression appears, accompanied by despair, and turns into apathy: the demoralisation syndrome: What's the point of even living?

Two dangers now threaten our system:

(a) Our guiding emotional mind is disorganised and confused, so that it can no longer give our body its proper instructions for living. Our normal body functions become disorganised as a result.

(b) This emotional mind may now also contain wrong instructions that can harm us by working actively against our well-being. Our disorganised functions become re-organised to work against our health.

Because our organism is born to cope, and has a practical mind to guide it in its coping, we have the need and the capacity for doing something useful and appropriate about any situation that we are in. Feeling fit means feeling capable, enabled, it is the feeling that we can come to grips with any situation, the feeling that we can assert ourselves in it. Feeling fit is a feeling that we can cope with the situation, even if it is difficult. We refer to this sense of fitness as feeling fighting fit.

Our practical-emotional mind is an arousing and guiding mind for coping with life: for coming to grips with the world that we inhabit, for keeping going, for staying alive in it. This mind also digests our experiences into useful memories, so that we may learn from them.

That is why we have a leading head with sense organs that prepare the world for us as a stage for our action, that make it into an arena for action, a playing field. That is also why we have arms for operating on this world, and legs for moving around in it. The only reason why we can and must perceive this world is because we must live from it, and to live from it, we must act on it. An organism must act, fight for its survival, and it can only do this if it feels fighting fit.

A situation may be easy for coping, or it may be difficult to deal with, but as long as it is only difficult, we are still coping somehow. When we are no longer coping, then this is no longer a normal, if difficult, situation. It has become an abnormal situation, a failure situation, a trap.

We now experience stress emotions: abnormal emotions that spell out our basic anger, anxiety, guilt, hopelessness, depression, and other such unbearable negative feelings of frustration.

This sense of frustration is what makes a trap intolerable.

Abnormal emotions are feelings that are no longer useful. They are no longer practical guides for living. They are no longer to be trusted because they may misguide us into believing that the situation is hopelessly lost.

If we cannot cope with the present situation, a difficult situation becomes closed off, and is now a trap. Then:

Coping is impossible: there is nothing I can do about it. Escaping is impossible: there is no opening for escape. Staying is impossible: a deep sense of frustration urges us to escape from the trap. Even an abnormal escape will now become acceptable: anything to get out of this intolerable situation. This decision is no voluntary choice: an abnormal escape route is prepared for our organism, without our conscious knowledge and consent.

Our everyday life is full of potential bodily and emotional traps for us, simply because our practical coping capacity has its normal human limits.

If we happen to fall into deep water and cannot swim, then we flail and flounder, we struggle desperately to stay afloat to breathe. If we can't manage to keep our head above the water, we drown, we sink helplessly, trapped in a situation with which we vainly try to cope.

We need not even be caged to feel trapped. Any situation that we cannot manage appropriately and effectively is a trap. Drowning is such a typical organismic trap, so is falling, and choking.

There are also emotional traps: situations that have happened but that we would rather have avoided, if we could. Whenever we feel angry or anxious during an event, we are trapped by this situation. What we experience is frustration, the frustration of our failure to cope.

Fortunately, not all traps are serious. Some are only minor embarrassments that do not last: we say something stupid and we feel acutely embarrassed, and remark that we could have bitten off our tongue, or that we wished we could have sunk through the floor, or fainted, or escaped this trap in some other way.

Major traps, however, have more serious consequences: these are situations in which our suffering is abnormal: too long and too strong, and this always means abnormal in quality. These may be desperately urgent situations, so that we experience an intense frustration that needs to be resolved, yet there is nothing we can do about it.

First we experience anger and anxiety, then depression, later followed by an abnormal resignation (apathy) or a flight into illness.

What we experience in the form of so many different abnormal emotions is a serious disorder, the sickness of a living being that is born to cope and that can no longer cope: a frustrated organism is a sick organism. This is an organism that will no longer have any reason to live if the entrapment is serious, and if it persists for too long. This is an illness that is as real as a pneumonia. We also need to recover from it, to heal, and to convalesce. Entrapment puts a strong damper on our life impulse.

EMOTIONAL FITNESS IS THE OPPOSITE OF STRESS

We are born with a sense of fitness which tells us that we are ready for action, for practical living, and for keeping alive. It means that we are, and feel, coping fit and fighting fit, that we are mentally free to fight.

We feel free to take an active hand in a situation, so that we can change it, if necessary, to our benefit. This is the total opposite of feeling trapped, hemmed in and powerless to do anything useful for ourselves.

Fitness is an expression of the dynamic life impulse itself. It primes us and directs us forward, towards the world that is happening in front of us, towards the future that is right now being made, and to which we naturally belong. It enables us, and invites us to take an active part in the making of the present.

Living organisms are always busy with the world that surrounds them, and this world is a reality of sights and sounds, and of smells and tastes, and of textures to feel. Living organisms are naturally interested in their fascinating environment of sights and sounds. Animals and young children are still locked into this spellbinding world of the senses, and cannot yet voluntarily escape it.

When a mother calls out to her child to come to the table, and the infant does not obey, it is not because it is naughty, but because it cannot hear and obey; its attention is being held elsewhere by a fascination with the situation. Its mother must shout loud enough to break this hypnotic spell.

Only adult human beings can break through this spell, and look away from this sensory world: to leave being in it, here and now, in order to think about it in its absence.

Human beings are otherwise no different from any other living organism; children have a natural and intense interest in the world that surrounds them and their interest is always accompanied by a sense of fitness and a willingness, even eagerness, to become involved with that world. Kids, we say, are brimming with energy, with the need for action, healthy and vigorous.

While we are healthy, we are interested in our surroundings, and we feel ready to interact with this world. We feel fit for doing things in it, such as eating and drinking, playing and working, making love, and so on.

The life impulse that is active in us expresses itself in this sense of fitness and interest; the future is open to us and we cope with our life. We have a sense of well-being that we take for granted. We don't walk around thumping our chests while telling everybody how well we feel, but we become aware of its absence when we are not well. How many times have we said, when we felt sick: 'I didn't realise how good it is to feel well, and to feel fit.'

But as soon as we feel well again, we quickly forget about our earlier unwellness, and we take our well-being and fitness for granted again. When we feel extra fit, we say that we are fighting fit, and this shows our readiness to come to grips with whatever situation comes along. What happens to these good feelings when we become stressed? We then lose our sense of well-being, our fitness and interest in the outside world, and we lose our appetite. These losses are often early signs that there is something wrong with our system.

The typical cancer patient may lose her or his appetite long before it can be blamed on the cancer. There was once an explanation that blamed it on toxins circulating in the body, which were supposed to have been produced by the cancer. However, the fact is that this loss of appetite disappears when the typical cancer patient stops being just that. It disappears as soon as the bad emotional software is extinguished and a more useful and positive programme has been installed.

Loss of appetite for food or other attractions is an early sign of a loss of interest in life itself, and that loss of interest is due to entrapment.

The statement: 'You have cancer and there is no effective treatment for it' is a typical entrapment situation. You want to be rid of this evil thing inside you, but there seems to be nothing you can concretely do. You can't get your hands on it, and you feel angry, and scared.

This dilemma is a result of the popular myth of the lay public: 'You are trapped with this deadly thing in your body, this monstrous thing, that grows in you, and that will soon eat into you and kill you, and there is nothing you can do about it'.

Isn't this precisely the horror theme of hopeless and helpless entrapment in the film *Aliens?*

The statement: 'You have cancer, but there is plenty you can do about it', refers to an altogether different situation, one that is not a trap. As long as you can do something about it, contribute usefully to it in some way, and never mind what way, you break this entrapment of your emotional mind. Kill the psychological cancer, and you increase your survival chances dramatically. Now you can begin the fight to overcome the biological cancer.

Chapter Thirteen

ENTRAPMENT AND HOPE

The stream that we call life is a very orderly process, and this orderliness is closely guarded by our regulating system. Stress is anything that disturbs this normal order so much that it can no longer right itself spontaneously and quickly.

If you stir a cup of tea, you create a little storm in it that gradually settles again. If you stir a living organism you create a disturbance that will be more quickly settled because there is an active self-righting system at work that will try to cancel out anything that disturbs the normal routine of a healthy life. This active self-righting is called regulation, and the system that performs that job, is called a regulating system. Sometimes the disturbance is so great, that it is too much for this self-righting system to handle. It will fail to restore the normal healthy order. The normal order has now made way for a dis-order, which is the state of stress.

We then say that this disturbance was too strong, that it was beyond our normal capacity for regulation: beyond our power for maintaining the normal order in our system. Our system is now disordered; it is no longer normally organised for living, but disorganised to a varying degree. A stressful event creates an excessive and abnormal disturbance, a disorder which we then experience emotionally and bodily as distress, as an illness of the organism.

THE THREE MAIN FORMS OF STRESS

There are minor stresses in life that come and go. We become a bit unsettled, so that we suffer a degree of disorganisation. But after a short while we regain our equilibrium, and life goes back to normal. This is just like a minor illness such as a cold. Our emotional mind has therefore successfully digested this experience, and even learned from it. This is one of its natural functions.

There are major stresses in life that are more unsettling, and that may take longer to settle. But even these will eventually ease so that we can cope again. We continue our life more or less as we lived it before, or perhaps pursue a different direction, but in either case we are back within our coping capacity.

Emotional stresses like these can be compared to more serious bodily illnesses such as a gall-bladder infection or pneumonia. It is important to remember this: psychological stress is equally an illness, from which we must recover and which requires time for convalescence. Just as it is impossible to recover immediately from pneumonia, it is not possible to be cured of stress in a day or two. The organism needs time to re-organise itself, to restore the normal practical order by self-regulation.

There is entrapment in life. This is the most serious form of stress. It leads to a profound disorganisation that may not be reversible, unless we refuse to remain trapped, and force our escape. In a trap, we are denied everything that we have been designed for, and that means, in short, freedom of action. This emotional trap is comparable to a body illness from which we do not recover. We remain an invalid.

We have been given, as our birthright, an ability to cope with life's situations, to adjust and to master and to gain some benefit from the situation for our survival first and for our enjoyment second.

Normally we cope with life. We move from one situation to the next so that we move through a series of situations towards a future of everapproaching new situations. We usually manage such situations; we cope so that we get something positive out of them for our survival or enjoyment.

This forward direction (or intentionality) of life continues like a steady stream of ever new and different situations. We live to cope with these, one new situation after another.

That coping ability is lost in an entrapment situation, and this current entrapment situation does not change, so that it continues without end. There is no future in it, and we are not doing what we were designed for. We are not managing it to our benefit and well-being. We are not coping.

This means that our organism is frustrated in all its natural directions and tendencies, and disorganised in all its natural functions. Nothing works normally, properly, any more.

If such entrapment continues, this disorganisation may become so severe that it is no longer compatible with life, unless we manage to rescue ourselves from it or allow ourselves to be freed with outside help. In the trap, we can no longer move from one situation to the next. The trap remains a trap. A trap is a situation that does not change, that does not move on. Our path forward is blocked. This intolerable present situation does not change. We cannot move freely, and we cannot grow further. We stagnate in the trap.

If we become resigned to staying in the trap, we give up hope that it will ever change, so that we give up life itself. Wild animals often die in such enduring captivity, and so do human beings who need their freedom of movement even more. There is no future in entrapment because the situation remains static and can no longer evolve normally. Without any hope of a future our emotional mind will die off. Even if our body remains alive we die emotionally because, without the freedom to move and grow, our emotional mind no longer has any reason to exist.

In such fatal resignation, we are thoroughly demoralised and apathetic. Our disorganisation is complete and our system is beyond regulation. It can no longer right itself. Regulation will now fail entirely, and death comes.

THE TWO SOURCES OF STRESS

Stress can come from outside situations that are imposed on us without involving our personality, or from a personality failure in an impossibly difficult situation.

Such externally caused stress situations are, for example, a bereavement, the loss of a job in bad economic times, civilian suffering in war, distress through natural disasters, and incarceration in concentration camps.

These conditions have nothing to do with our personality which is the personal part of our emotional mind. They are states or situations that would stress anybody.

Sometimes, however, the distress comes from a failure to cope that originates in our individual personality. Someone else may be able to escape a trap that proves too much for our specific personality. This represents an internal trap, as it were, in contrast to the external traps described above. This internal trap is a private and personal trap, a trap in our personal existence from which we cannot escape, held back by an oversensitive conscience or emotional inadequacy.

Such personal entrapment may lead to a quiet despair that is as deep as it is silent. We despair because there is no future in our trap, and there seems no future in continuing to live. We are very unhappy with our life as it is, but we can't bring ourselves to do anything about it. We don't move forward, and we don't grow.

We may then have no choice but to continue to live our life as a dull routine, automatically, helplessly, without hope and without interest. One goes through the meaningless motions for the sake of appearances. This kind of living is like existing in an internal concentration camp.

HOPELESSNESS IN ENTRAPMENT

Life is a stream. It is a forward movement into an always open immediate future. This present situation always goes over into the next present one, the morning changes into afternoon, and today flows into tomorrow. Life grows. It is directed towards a future, to the situation which comes next.

Life is always going somewhere, and this somewhere is always in the future. Our bodily needs show this very clearly: hunger implies that we shall soon eat, sleepiness promises sleep, and so on. A need is a sensation that implies a future fulfilment.

If you block this forward-looking stream, its movement stops, and life becomes a stagnant pool that begins to breed disease. In living systems nothing can stand still: stagnation means breakdown. If there is no future in being alive here and now, this life will become stagnant in apathy, and it may soon stop altogether.

In depression, the future looks narrow and dim: it looks bleak and miserable so that, with such an outlook, people will turn naturally back towards the past. But as long as there is some future, no matter how bleak it may appear to be right now, the future will still be open, and life continues.

It is when this future disappears from view entirely that the depressed patient will begin to self-destruct, by committing suicide or by regulation failure (dysregulation).

As long as there is a future in any difficult situation, even if it is a faint glimmer of one, life can continue its forward movement. When we look at it from an emotional point of view, we call this openness of the future: hope. When we view it biologically, we could call this same openness of the future the natural growth direction of all living systems.

Biologically, living systems are called open systems. They are open to the world, from which they must constantly take food and fuel and excrete back what they don't need.

This openness also implies a being open to the future, because our impatient needs are all future-directed sensations. Living systems, when they are not recuperating from activities, are alert and ready for change, primed and fit for coping with the coming situation.

There is only one situation in life in which this future will be closed off, and that is in entrapment. A trap is a place, a condition, or an emotional situation, that offers no hope of escape. You are in it, and you cannot get out of it. But you can't stay in it either, because a trap is an unbearable state of frustration, like the feeling that you can't breathe any more, or the feeling that you are bursting apart with great anger, or cringing and shrivelling in intense anxiety. It can also be the intolerable feeling that you are locked in with some dreadful disease.

We gave a quick summary of the stages of entrapment in the previous chapter. Let us now take a closer look at some of these.

Second stage of entrapment. This phase is filled with anger and anxiety, with a strong sense of rebellion: 'This can't be happening to me'. It brings a frustration that compels us to search for means of escape.

Frustration is that desperate feeling that you can't stand this situation any more, that anything is better than continuing with it. But it is also the feeling that there is absolutely nothing you can do about it.

We use statements such as: it makes me mad just to think about it, and: he drives me crazy with his problems, when we want to express this intolerable state of sheer frustration. It is like an itch we are not allowed to scratch: it drives us up the wall.

There are relatively minor emotional traps in our daily life, as we said before, such as embarrassment, for example. We have said something stupid or hurtful, and we are mortified. This means we are trapped, that we cannot undo the situation, don't know what to do about it, and wish only to escape from it. Our mood, the indicator of our vitality, has an oppressive quality. When the trap opens, we feel relieved of this burdened feeling and we can breathe freely again. If the trap is more serious, then this wish grows into an intense need to escape. We may experience escape fantasies, wishing we were elsewhere, far away.

In a major entrapment situation, our emotional mind looks for a means of escape that may no longer be practical, such as a flight into illness, a fugue with amnesia, or suicide. This kind of escape is now no longer something that we can control. It is out of our hands, it just happens to us.

Third stage of entrapment. This begins when our sense of rebellion and restless frustration disappear, and give way to resignation in quiet despair. We have now lost all hope of escaping. Our attempts have been in vain, and we are ready to give up trying. We resign ourselves to continuing entrapment if we cannot even find an abnormal escape route. This is when we begin the road to self-destruction. We now become demoralised, apathetic and helpless. We lose all interest in life, because we have lost all hope.

The previously open future is now closed off to us, so that we begin to languish and wither. We may even die an unnecessary death unless someone will come to our rescue, because we can now no longer help ourselves. We may drift slowly, or even more rapidly, into a psychogenic death.

The fate of animals that are caged, and cannot adapt to their captive state, is a typical biological example of such a major entrapment. Their first reaction is frustration (which humans would experience as anger and anxiety). They pace restlessly around the fence, whining while they search vainly for an escape route.

When frustration mounts, they may jump blindly and recklessly at the fence, hurting themselves in the process, but whatever they try, using (by now disordered) instincts and emotions, it is all in vain. They now lose what humans call hope, that vital biological ingredient for living.

Abnormal resignation now overcomes them. They lose interest and lie down listlessly, no longer responsive to the natural calls of their animal world. They do not mate, they languish, and may eventually stop eating and drinking, and die from this apathy.

If they don't die, they lie about, occasionally roused from their lethargy by some unusual sound, or by food, but that is all. The mild excitement is soon over, and they sink back into their usual torpid state. We may well say that they are now no longer really alive, in the sense that this is not the natural life of a free living animal. They lead a useless vegetable existence. Functionally, as free-living animals that are born to cope, they have already died.

We are not all that different from animal organisms when we are trapped, even if we express this entrapment in other, typically human, ways.

Typical emotional examples in humans come from experiences in concentration camps and prisoner of war camps. Those who lost hope died prematurely. This was known as give-up-itis and it was typically a situation of total demoralisation: of helpless despair, of lost hope, and of absence of human support. Apathy comes and the organism withers. It does not want to eat or drink, and dies.

Other examples come from the type of death that is known as a psychogenic or psychosomatic death. This happens when a person is emotionally trapped in a situation in which some tribal law has been broken. A curse is placed on this person, who now proceeds to die in the same mysterious manner as caged animals and prisoners. In Australia there is the ancient and powerful Aboriginal practice of bone-pointing; a tribal punishment by cursing that leads to a psychogenic death. This self-produced death is known elsewhere as voodoo death, and it comes about in the same manner.

Socially assisted dying. If we look at this bone-pointing (or voodoo) death, we may also observe that there is an additional problem, namely that the entire social environment of the victim of the curse is involved in helping him to die. This emotional situation is thus closed for him, and becomes a complete trap. No matter where he goes, he will be reminded by his social environment that he is expected to die. He can't escape.

And this is precisely the kind of emotional situation that the typical cancer patient, the cancer-voodoo victim, may find herself or himself trapped in.

Mr TCP expects himself to die, because he believes that he must die and his social environment contributes to his wrong belief, by having, and by showing him, the same expectation. 'Everybody around me reminds me of it, and I remind myself of it every moment that I am awake, and I wish that I could just turn my mind off, stop it in some way. I meet friends and they show a sorrowful face when they see me. I go to the doctor and he will look serious, I look at my wife, and I can see the grief and pity on her face. Everybody seems to have given me up'.

Can there be any doubt that this patient feels well and truly trapped, he feels that he has no option but to die, and he despairingly feels that his social environment helps him into the grave?

HOPE IS NOT A PSYCHOLOGICAL LUXURY

Hope is a fundamental part of the life impulse itself. It is a biological part of the openness of our living substance to the sensory world around it. Hope is part of our biological make-up as living organisms. It is a biological necessity because it gives us an option, an alternative to dying.

When we are thirsty, we hope to drink soon and if we are ill, we hope to recover. We take this hope, this confidence in our future, for granted. Hope is a biological openness to the future.

Otherwise why would a lion bother to stalk its prey? Why would a cat jump from a fence on to the roof, if not in the taken-for-granted and confident hope that it will succeed?

Why should we summon the motivation and energy to get up in the morning, and to try anything, if it were not based on the expectation of making it through the day, of achieving what we want? This hope may be taken for granted, but it is always there and is more like a confidence in the future than a wish for it. Hope is the forward direction of the life impulse that always faces the immediate future. The future is reality that is just now coming into being, and we expect it to come as usual.

Without a possible future there is no hope, and we become like a condemned person who is marked for execution, without hope of a last minute reprieve.

That we take hope for granted in our daily affairs, means it is a fundamental part of our life. It never occurs to us to doubt it. Every time we swallow food we take it for granted that it will go down the proper tube, and not land in our lungs. It could go wrong, of course, just as it is possible (but very unlikely) that a stone will not fall but go up instead, or that the sun may not rise tomorrow. Life aims at surviving. The probability of normal surviving is greater than that of untimely dying, or no life would be possible. Hope is precisely this greater probability for survival.

Taking away hope is not merely a psychological disappointment, it is the removal of our biological faith in a future. It is a bad, even fatal, mistake. Remove hope completely and you douse the life impulse itself by taking away the motive for its continuation.

Block a living being's future, and it no longer has any reason to live. Its forward growth into an open future is paralysed. It must wilt and lose its life in the stagnant apathy of entrapment. Removing hope amounts to blocking the stream of life. It stops flowing.

Apathy means feelinglessness, a total loss of interest, and of natural openness towards the world. It is a loss of all that is dynamic in life. A loss of all feeling makes normal movement almost impossible. As long as there is hope, there is a possibility for useful action, for doing something about a situation, for coming to grips with it. As long as there is hope, the situation is not yet a trap, merely a difficult situation that can still be overcome.

We are designed and built to behave usefully in our life, to be reasonably effective, and fit to act. We take the hope that is implied in this capacity for living for granted. The expectation that we do have a future is our motive power for stirring ourselves into action. Without it, why should we bother to do anything at all? A melancholic patient lies in a stupor, unable and unmotivated to move, because the future is no longer open to her organism.

Take away hope and you take away the biological reason for being alive. This is what that expression give-up-itis means. It is a potentially fatal paralysis of our biological need to survive and demonstrates clearly how severe the disorganisation of our system is.

Dr Engel wrote about the combination of hopelessness and helplessness; the feelings of helplessness and hopelessness are the signs of the greatest degree of disorganisation. These tell us that there is a mood of giving up, a feeling that it is impossible to carry on, to cope with the stress, and that it is all too much. There is a sense of despair and futility, a feeling that there is nothing left (*Psychological Development in Health and Disease*, page 174).

By giving up the struggle for freedom when we find ourselves in an entrapment situation, we lose interest in finding a proper way out: 'What's the use, and what does it matter anyway?' This loss of interest is a loss of appetite for living. The loss of appetite for food is often the first sign of giving up the fight for freedom. This is usually followed by the loss of interest in sexual activity, then in doing things for oneself. The world of interests shrinks gradually until it is only a little circle centred around this fitless and apathetic body.

A loss of appetite for food can appear early, too early to be accounted for by the illness induced by the biological cancer (assuming that this is not caused by chemotherapy). It is produced by the psychological cancer instead, and it can be overcome by ceasing to be a typical cancer patient.

What does this loss of appetite mean? It is not simply that we don't want to eat, but it is an inability to eat. A typical statement is: 'I can't bring myself to eat, the food won't go down'. This sign indicates a profound disorganisation of our system, that the regulation of life itself has been affected. It is the stagnation of the most basic of our living functions in entrapment, and it is this inability that leads to such an early loss of appetite and weight. The need to take in food or drink is the second most powerful need of our organism. The newborn baby breathes as its first vital compulsion to live, then drinks as the second most urgent instinct for living. The infant who ceases to drink is a seriously ill organism, because he or she may stop breathing next.

The return of appetite is a good sign because it indicates the waking up of the life impulse, as every experienced doctor and nurse well knows. It is the welcome reawakening of the *vis medicatrix naturae* in us, that was asleep in apathy before.

Apart from unusual circumstances, such as physical captivity during war, entrapment is for the human being an entrapment in emotional situations, and this is what we are going to examine next.

There are people who advise that a cancer patient must come to terms with the cancer, and face the dismal prospect of dying openly and courageously. These people are very rarely patients themselves. It is always easier to expect someone else to be brave.

We must suspect this attitude if it comes early in the course of the illness, because it is the typical cancer patient who often puts up this false bravado.

We must look into it to make sure that it is real and deeply felt. If so, this mind is set, and cannot, and perhaps should not, be changed.

Must Mr TCP accept death before it is absolutely inevitable? And when is death ever absolutely inevitable before the very moment that it actually happens? Should he say goodbye before he must go? Is this advice itself not a form of bone-pointing?

Part Four

HEALING

Chapter Fourteen

INTRODUCTION TO HEALING

When we look at the way cancer patients react to the diagnosis and relate this reaction to the eventual outcome of the disorder, we see that they fall into two large groups. One group is what we may call a do better group. The other the do not (so) well group.

The do better group. It has now become generally recognised and accepted that this group consists of persons who have a different response to the diagnosis and the illness. I find it to be particularly true for the first six months or so after the diagnosis. In this group we find people who respond with the following typical coping style (the expressions in italics indicate how that has been described in various psychosomatic investigations).

- They adopt a *fighting spirit* or *fighting attitude.*
- They are able to *externalise their hostility and anger.*
- They have *decreased levels of anxiety and depression.*
- This group has been found to have a *significantly higher* survival rate.

Children appear to belong to this group. They cope better with the diagnosis, perhaps partly because they do not realise the significance that the diagnosis of cancer has for the adult.

That patients with a fighting spirit do better is nothing new or surprising. The medical world seems to have largely forgotten that, in its preoccupation with advanced medical techniques. In older medical texts from before the Second World War, this good spirit of the patient was a favourable prognostic indicator, meaning that the patient had a better chance of recovery, in spite of the relatively primitive therapeutic arsenal in those days. A positive attitude, this determination to get well, was regarded as being important then, and it is still so now and particularly if there is no specific and effective medical treatment available.

The do not (so) well group. This group consists of people who respond differently to the diagnosis; the difference appearing to lie in the absence of a fighting spirit. It is therefore no wonder that there is an increased risk of early suicide in this group.

Some persons respond with a sense of despair, helplessness and hopelessness to the diagnosis. Instead of the fighting spirit, they show a giving-up attitude right from the start. The poor attitude amounts to a silent consent to the illness, be it cancer or any other kind of infection. There is little resistance, little rebellion, and no rejection. This emotional sickness must always be regarded as a serious complication of the cancerous infection.

Others show what has been described as a stoic attitude, of calm acceptance. This sounds better than it really is; it is not a rational and emotionally neutral acceptance of having cancer. Nobody is that good. Instead, this attitude is an unresisting acceptance of a death sentence. The emotional mind is so locked up, so trapped, that it cannot rebel. It is difficult for many such persons to open their mind to the freedom to rebel and fight, because the death sentence seems to have been accepted with total certainty. Although such persons may appear calm on the surface, this almost delusional certainty points to a serious disorganisation of their emotional mind.

Their emotional mind refuses to shift from its rigid position. When these persons begin psychotherapy, they soon drop out unchanged and unconvinced, doomed by their own delusion that death is inevitable. Their emotional mind is so tightly clenched that they are incapable of seeing any option but death.

The stoic has an inner pride, an inner stiffness that will not allow him or her to cause trouble for others. There is a strong inner inhibition against being difficult. This person's environment may play the game, and everything may seem under control on the surface. Everyone politely ignores the illness, and the unnatural silence of course only emphasises it.

Looking at this do not so well group, we may now realise where the trouble really lies. These are the TCPs, those typical cancer patients who feel trapped by 'that cancer, which to me means death', as one patient put it. Consider the following points:

(a) The bereavement (loss) that has often been described in the literature, and which is supposed to precede the diagnosis of clinical cancer, is not always present. Moreover, there is sometimes no evidence of any other crisis situation in the recent past that could have been responsible.

Instead, a more enduring condition is often present, a silent stress condition that has been left unacknowledged. This is a state of quiet despair about an unhappy and unsatisfactory life that one cannot change. This condition is the entrapment of the emotional mind.

The chronic discontent does not cause cancer, but it may promote its growth by reducing the general efficiency of regulation.

(b) The early suicide rate points clearly to a sense of being trapped by the myth of an unstoppable, growing cancer inside one's body.

(c) The response of despair, depression and hopelessness is another indication of this condition of emotional entrapment; these are the signs of being trapped and giving up. We may see this in two situations, as we have said:

(i) In an entrapment by life before the diagnosis of cancer; a serious personal emotional entrapment situation.

(ii) In an entrapment with death, brought about by a belief in the myth of an inevitable death by cancer; the 'voodoo curse' of the diagnosis of clinical cancer.

(d) There is little fighting spirit in this group, little of that positive attitude that characterises the do-better group. This poor coping style is a self-repressive manner of self management. It is based on a self-denying and self-sacrificing attitude, that tells us a sense of adequate self-worth is lacking.

Sometimes death is the preferred route out of an emotional dilemma that seems to be too difficult to solve, so that there is a private consent to it. It is sometimes easier to die than to live on. One patient seemed eager to do everything possible to survive, yet all his enthusiasm lacked conviction. When I asked him about this, he was silent for a while, and then admitted that it would really be easier for him if he were to die. His family situation had become a trap, too difficult to solve, so that death was the preferred option. He died.

The self-image of 'I am not good enough' is one reason for the state of mind: 'There is nothing much I can do to help myself and I give up'. This kind of thinking tells us that there is a resignation to entrapment which appears early and too easily in the fight.

The do better group consists of those who, on finding themselves trapped with cancer, refuse to resign themselves to being trapped with the myth of the inevitability of death. They reject the possibility and feel motivated to take up the challenge. They are assertive rather than helpless, and rebellious rather than depressed and despairing.

What has been described as anger or hostility in this do better group, is typically a rebellious fighting spirit which is lacking in the other group. The rebellious attitude implies a rejection: 'I am not going to submit to the cancer, I refuse to accept it, I'll fight my way out of this situation somehow'. This is the exact opposite of the attitude of giving up.

Finding ourselves emotionally trapped and resigning ourselves to entrapment are two entirely different things. Becoming aware of the trap should lead to a determined effort to break out of this existential trap, before the cancer grows to a clinical cancer. In this way we can avoid the psychosomatic death-trap after the diagnosis.

The private-personal trap may disorganise our regulating system to such a degree that it promotes cancer growth. We may find we are trapped by life, meaning that we are stuck in a situation in which we suffer and we cannot get out of because we haven't got the right personality for escaping. This is a chronic emotional illness, and we need help.

The psychosomatic death trap is the voodoo curse, the myth that death is inevitable. This is a trap that begins after the diagnosis. It is an acute emotional illness and requires urgent treatment. We may already be resigned to a personal emotional trap with life which has sapped our strength to resist. We now find ourselves in a second trap: a trap with death.

THE VOODOO TRAP

It takes courage and determination to reject both the medical and social bone-pointing behaviour. Too many people, including the medical staff involved in the treatment, seem to have the faulty attitude (even if it is never expressed) that all cancer patients must sooner or later die from it, barring miracles.

Patients who have been alerted to this bone-pointing behaviour in the medical staff should recognise it, and can either learn to ignore it or bring the bad attitude to the notice of the persons concerned.

Obliquely or openly, our environment generally expects the cancer patient to die from the cancer. The frightened Mr TCP, who has already been brought into a hypnosis-like state by his high anxiety, may now meet such life-destroying hypnotic attitudes and suggestions everywhere. Consider this scene, for example. It contains a suggestion to Mr TCP who has been made all too ready for it by his anxiety: 'You are going to be very nauseated from this chemotherapy, Mr TCP, so we'll give you a big dose of Maxolon to ease it and stop your vomiting.'

How can Mr TCP now possibly escape being nauseated? This suggestion has come from someone in authority, such as the doctor or nursing sister. Such wrong hypnotic suggestions can make symptoms needlessly worse.

Mr TCP has become highly sensitised and is emotionally allergic to many uncalled for remarks, to statements which are unnecessary, and made inadvertently. Yet, we would not think of spraying an asthmatic who is allergic to dust mite, with a dose of it. Mr TCP is allergic to pessimistic expressions because they cause him days of suffering.

As far as the medical profession is concerned, such suggestive aggravation is poor medicine, even if the attitude is taken to be realistic. People do become nauseated, and they do lose their hair with certain therapies, but they should only have to suffer those symptoms that are unavoidable.

There is a big difference between the powerfully suggestive and authoritarian: 'You will suffer this side effect', and the milder caution: 'You may suffer this side effect'. 'You will' does not offer any alternative, whereas 'you may' implies that he may not develop the side effect. In the language of hypnosis, it means he does not absolutely have to suffer the side effect.

From a medical-biological point of view, clinical cancer is a complication of the earlier infection, brought about by poor resistance to alien invasion. Pneumonia may complicate a viral upper respiratory tract infection for the same reason, but few people are prepared to say that such a patient is doomed.

If someone dies from viral pneumonia, everyone is horrified. 'What a thing to happen, what bad luck, who would have thought that such a thing was possible'. It is so unexpected that it takes everybody by surprise. Yet Mr TCP has to endure the powerful voodoo of dying in a social conspiracy which everybody joins.

Everyone, doctors included, should view cancer as we view any other serious infection. Many immunologists have said cancer belongs to the large class of infections, and this makes good biological sense.

Even if a doctor believes the cancer is a fatal disorder, this is the wrong attitude to take to the patient who has the job of trying to survive it. To say to Mr TCP that his cancer is fatal, will make him believe he is now doomed. He will expect to die because he experiences what the doctor says as a voodoo curse. The doctor may even believe that he is giving Mr TCP the objective truth. But the patient cannot grasp that objective prognosis as a neutral truth. He hears a voodoo curse. What was meant as a prediction based on statistics, a mere likelihood, will be accepted by Mr TCP as the certainty of dying.

It is a poor doctor who transmits to the patient feelings that imply: 'I am trying to treat you, but understand that you may be a hopeless case. Unless a miracle happens, you're very likely going to die from this.'

Illness, said Professor Frank, often produces a vicious circle by creating [negative] emotions that aggravate it (page 47).

Some readers may think that such examples of negative hypnotic instruction are exaggerated. However, years of experience in supportive therapy in general practice have made me aware of how badly informed specialists and other staff can be in their psychological approach to vulnerable cancer patients. The nursing staff, to their considerable credit, are generally more positively supportive and open to the emotional side of the cancer problem than the doctors.

The difference between being frankly open and being callous may be so small that it requires some discernment to perceive it. What is often explained as only being realistic, can be so traumatic that patients say they feel sick for days or weeks afterwards. How can such trauma ever be justified, when the Hippocratic oath demands that anything we do must not hurt the patient?

Let me repeat that if someone has the unspoken attitude of: 'I expect you to die', it will be strongly felt by Mr TCP. Imagine the impact that such an attitude must have on a highly sensitised

Mr TCP, when everybody around him unknowingly transmits it to him. It is like a hay-fever sufferer caught in a pollen-rich environment.

A socially enacted voodoo curse has a powerful effect on Mr TCP, even if he is not aware of it. He loses weight as his appetite fades; he languishes, and feels depressed and desperate. His emotional mind has got the message, even if his rational mind still knows nothing about all this.

There appears to be a clear correlation between a rebellious attitude and a better outcome. People who openly express their discontent are not prepared to accept defeat easily, and they are not typical cancer patients. They are those fighters with a positive attitude, people who refuse to accept the social voodoo.

Chapter Fifteen

MORE ABOUT HEALING

If we wish to eliminate the negative attitude, we must first know where it can be found. Wrong expectations may occur among treating doctors and other medical staff, in the social environment of family and friends, and finally (and most importantly) in ourselves.

When this needless psychological complication (an unwelcome emotional disorder) has been removed from our emotional mind, we can then use the unburdened mind to concentrate on the biological complication of cancer, and explore the ways in which we can best assist mother nature in her effort to heal us. This will also assist oncologists in their attempt to eradicate or control the biological cancer.

DEHYPNOTISATION

Mr TCP must be relieved of the voodoo curse that has captured and occupied his emotional mind. This may be done even when he is treated with chemotherapy or radiotherapy. How should he do it?

(a) He himself must know quite clearly about the existence of this curse, and realise that it is based on a mistaken belief. Mr TCP must then learn to relax and visualise for himself a countering positive attitude.

(b) His medical and social environment must also become aware of it. This strategy is not just optional, it is crucial. The curse of a witch doctor may not work well if it is not supported by the rest of the tribe. We may have the strength to resist the idea of cancer leading inevitably to death, if our social environment does not cooperate by bone-pointing us. We shall do even better if they support us, by encouraging us to fight for our recovery. A subtle form of bone-pointing may arise, quite unintentionally, if the family now wants to spend quality time with Mr TCP.

Even in the hospital environment Mr TCP may become exposed to bone-pointing by the medical staff. Some staff members may be motivated by nervousness in dealing with him, others by a need to be open and frank. In both cases Mr TCP may suffer. Here is an example from a patient's experience: a nursing sister comes to have a little chat with him before his treatment starts: 'You were told not to expect too much from this, weren't you? No? Didn't the doctor tell you? He doesn't think that you have much chance, unfortunately.'

Another example: his surgeon tells Mr TCP that he has only a poor chance of recovery, and says kindly: 'Go home, Mr TCP and enjoy every day'. Implied in this well-meant advice is the statement: 'You haven't got much time left, Mr TCP, so that every day that you are alive is a bonus.'

This is pure bone-pointing. Each passing day will now serve to bring the dreaded end closer. Mr TCP will find it impossible to enjoy his days with that hanging over him and the days will be like the ticking of a vital clock until the appointed time arrives.

Other medical staff are more sensitive and yet practical. They will treat Mr TCP as if he had an ordinary infectious complication which may be serious, but not necessarily fatal: 'It is serious, Mr TCP, but you'll fight it, won't you. We'll do our best to help you get over this.'

They will also encourage him to take an active part in his own recovery. It is this deep need for taking an active part in their own healing, that drives people to alternative forms of treatment which offer the possibility.

It is not usually given by conventional medicine because it prefers its patients to remain passive and helpless. The person becomes a mere patient.

TWO QUESTIONS

Two questions need to be answered at this point:

    (i) Does this supportive attitude mean being dishonest?

    (ii) Does this supportive attitude really help Mr TCP?

Can it really make a difference to the success or failure of his treatment, whether Mr TCP accepts that he is terminal or whether he is determined to live? How can this difference in attitude possibly influence biological cancer?

In fairness to medical practitioners it must be said that although the threat of legal complications does promote a more careful medical practice, the legal system also acts against good practice.

Doctors get into medico-legal trouble if they don't test, and into trouble from the government if they do test. To have to discern under pressure between what is enough, and what is too little or too much, can stress the weary medical brain considerably.

The main reason for the harsh attitude of so many doctors in giving their opinion to patients whom they don't know well enough, seems to be the fear of legal complications. To cover themselves, therefore, many doctors predict the worst possible outcome. If things go well from here, nobody is (hopefully) going to complain about getting well again, and we can always call it a miracle. If not, then nobody can say that he or she was not clearly warned.

This is important for the emotional well-being of Mr TCP, so let us look a little more closely at this worst possible prognosis: nobody can ever predict that an illness is fatal, because that is claiming to be able to foretell the future. There is an enormous difference between saying that an illness is fatal for the average statistical person, and that it may be fatal for you, the unpredictable unique individual.

Many people are still around in spite of average predictions because these do not take into account the person who has the illness, and how this unique individual responds to the illness. How such a person reacts to the statement must influence the course of the illness in some way. Such personal input is a factor in the equation that may be minor or major, but it can never be ignored. This personal factor does not enter the statistics, of course. Yet it would be reasonable to expect the type of personality to be included, together with the type of cancer, and the type of treatment.

As one patient, mentioned earlier, said to her surgeon: 'Doctor, you may know your statistics, but you don't know me'. And I could not put this more simply and correctly. Once alerted to the presence of the bowel cancer, she absolutely refused (she said) to consider the possibility that a cancer could grow inside her own body.

And when I said that she had become 'a spontaneous remission' without any treatment, she snorted: 'Spontaneous remission nothing! No, I didn't allow it to grow.' With such remarks, this lady taught me more than I could have taught her.

She expected to win the fight, and she did. Such spontaneous remissions are probably not so much rare as rarely recognised. Is this so strange that we should expect to win? Does this not characterise our practical and healthy mind? People gamble. Why should they, if they don't expect to win? We take chances all the time, even when we eat, or cross the road, but we don't expect to fail.

Students of physics may believe that statistical averages also apply in the reality of living beings, but Mother Nature says: 'No, not in my world.' The science of statistics, like that of mathematics, is a human invention, a clever thinking tool with which the scientist hopes to understand something of a complex reality. He or she gets a statistical picture of it, but never the reality itself. Reality and its statistical version are never the same thing, just as a person and her portrait are not the same.

Imagine four people playing poker: Father Physics assures us that each player has an equal chance of getting good cards, if they all play long enough. Mother Chaos says: Ha, just watch me: I'll make person A always get good cards, and deal person B consistently bad cards, so that B will always hate to play. Father Physics will then say that he has no influence over the fate of individual cases, while other players console person B with the old saying: unlucky at cards, but lucky in love.

Every single individual card game shows hands that are against all odds: four aces may come up three or four times in a poker session, and usually with the same people, and the calculated odds against this happening are staggering.

Nature does not work according to theoretical statistics. She follows the patterns of chaos instead. Statistical odds should not be taken too seriously in life, because they are accurate as predictions, as far as they go, but for very large groups. Such statistics are not useful in the much smaller numbers of our practical individual daily life, or no gambling would be possible, and games and sports would never have been invented.

Individual daily life is ruled, not by statistics, but by a highly creative uncertainty that appears everywhere as the unexpected, as a surprise event. Can we ever know for certain what the next hour will bring? Never, because there is creative uncertainty at work which may show itself in the crevice between what we usually and routinely expect, and what can actually happen.

We may do our technical best, but we realise that there is always a gap between our best effort and the hoped for result. While scientists use statistics specifically to cover that gap of fundamental uncertainty, other human beings pray to their fate-determining god or use superstitious rituals to influence it. The gap of uncertainty belongs to the creative gods of chaos. In this gap, anything is possible that is not possible in a rational system.

This unpredictable gap represents a hope that can never be removed from our living reality. It is the very essence of reality.

The gods of chaos say: nothing is certain before the moment it concretely and actually happens. And we listen and accept.

It makes an enormous difference to his psychological and even biological healing, if Mr TCP can reject being an invalid and works on himself to become fighting fit. This insight is as old as medicine itself, and it was the basis for therapy long before the use of medicines and surgery.

This fighting spirit is what every doctor likes to see in a patient, because no disorder can affect our organism without involving both body and emotional mind. Body and mind do not exist outside each other as separate entities. The body is contained in the emotional mind, as we have seen. This is why a positive attitude supports bodily healing while a negative one works for the illness. Let me repeat, you have no choice: if you don't actively assist healing, then you automatically work against it. There is no such thing as being neutral where your own health is concerned.

A soldier (assuming a male) at the front has to be motivated to fight. When we speak about front-line morale, this means that both his body and emotional mind must be geared to winning the fight. The battle has not yet been decided, but each side is fighting in the expectation of winning.

If the soldier is being encouraged to fight, and is stimulated to a maximum fighting capacity by concerted encouragement, is such aiming to win the fight dishonest? We are not talking about the absurd extremes of war propaganda, but of an appeal to the soldier to mobilise his resources, and to do his best to defend his country.

A fighting fit soldier has a fighting spirit, is well motivated, and is in a good nutritional state. His emotional and physical well-being is of the highest importance if the war is to be won. As so many recent wars have shown, morale is equal to superior manpower and technology. Can we say as much for cancer sufferers, especially those who are demoralised?

Demoralisation is a disease of the emotional mind. The battle against psychological cancer is a fight against an unnecessary voodoo death. A voodoo death is a death by fright and a death by despair. It is not an understandable reaction to the idea of having cancer: Mr TCP is emotionally ill and this illness is as real and as serious as a bout of meningitis. Mr TCP needs urgent psychological help.

The presence of the biological cancer is already an indication of lowered resistance against foreign invasion. The voodoo curse is a new foreign invasion, a mental invasion, that finds easy acceptance in Mr TCP's emotional mind. Already his mind is suffering from a lack of emotional resistance against alien invasion.

The voodoo curse (he must die) invades his emotional mind and takes increasing hold of it until it occupies his mind completely. If Mr TCP is convinced: 'I must die because my condition is hopeless', the belief will disorganise his whole organism even further. His regulating system has to work harder and the regulating system itself will become disorganised.

If the regulating system itself now begins to suffer, it can no longer perform its function of maintaining life. It is now no longer a matter of losing well-being, but of losing life.

If Mr TCP dies a voodoo death, the disorder that exists in his emotional mind and body (and created by his demoralised state) has been too much for his organism to cope with. This severe disorganisation would paralyse his life-supporting and life-maintaining regulating systems.

What is demoralisation? In becoming demoralised, we become an organism without hope and without purpose. Our mind can no longer guide our practical organism towards the open future.

The state of demoralisation is itself a severe illness that may be fatal. This emotional disorder is a separate condition from the original biological cancer. The hypnotised emotional mind begins to issue orders that are contrary to the normally beneficial running of the system, and the confused regulating system sends self-destructive dis-orders through to lower levels of regulation. These lower levels can only obey those abnormal orders from higher up.

A complete disorganisation of the system is the result. This disorganisation is such a severe disorder that it is no longer compatible with maintaining the orderly function that we call life.

Chapter Sixteen

HEALING FROM THE
PSYCHOLOGICAL CANCER

LIFE AND LOGIC

Life is an orderly process; our tissues and organs form a strictly law-abiding and orderly community, a healthy living order. This living order is not a rational order, however, it does not run according to rational logic.

Mother Nature herself does not work on the basis of rational logic. Don't we know this from experience? Where is the logic of an innocent child suffering? Where is the logic of having to defend oneself from human and other biological enemies? Rational logic is simple and transparent; even a computer can work with it. Emotional logic, on the other hand, is always complex. It may sometimes be crude and harsh (an eye for an eye), but it is always complicated, as any attempt at analysis will show. Emotional logic may be so subtle and sophisticated that it can baffle our rational-intellectual mind. We then call this emotional logic chaotic or capricious.

We cannot always find rational logic in our living reality because this brand of logic is a human invention. Sometimes we can apply it to our situation, but more often we cannot. The bitter cry of: 'Why? Why did it have to happen? Why me? I've never done anything bad on purpose. Where is the sense of it?' is something that we are all familiar with. It means we are trying to look for a logical reason in the wrong place. The problem is well illustrated in the biblical story of Job, which has been aptly called the first existentialist writing.

We always seem to expect reality to follow the same rational pattern that we think in intellectually, and we are generally disappointed in this expectation. Emotional mathematics is usually too complicated for our rational mind to understand because it works with diffuse qualities, and not with clearly defined quantities.

Life itself is outside rational explanations, and many scientists have gone through contortions of thinking to explain why life can exist against all rational odds. A Dutch scientist once calculated that our rational idea of an accidental biochemical origin of life is so unlikely, that we might as well throw some matches in the air, and expect them to come down as the word life. Some religions claim that their concept of God produced life on earth, and some scientists even claim two gods whom they call 'time' and 'chance' to explain the same evolution.

It is not the place here to start talking about the origin of life, and I only wish to point this out: don't be too fussed about whether or not some belief or visual image that you want to work with is rational or not. It does not have to be rationally possible to be effective.

What is real is whatever is effective, and never mind if this is against rational logic. It is rational logic that is more likely to be useless, and therefore wrong. Give an asthmatic smoker all the rational reasons in the world to stop smoking, and see how useless that is. We live in an age in which rationality is rapidly losing its respectability in such sciences as phenomenological psychology and modern physics (quantum theory).

If, according to rational logic, some event should not happen, it does not mean that it is impossible, it only means it would never happen if reality ran according to rational logic. But even inanimate physical reality is not such a rational order, let alone the reality of living. The order of life is simply too complex to be rational. The rationally impossible is emotionally possible.

What is real for the emotional mind may be fiction and fantasy for the rational mind; yet, which affects us? A monster from outer space makes us break out in a panic during a nightmare, but who has ever drooled about Einstein's theory of relativity or wheezed on hearing of the law of causality?

Whatever moves us, what affects us, and changes our organism in some way: that is real. The practical definition of our reality is this: reality is that which works on our system, which affects us. Whether or not that reality accords with a rational order means nothing.

This is a common effect in hypnosis, where the touch of a cool pencil can cause a burn if burning is suggested to and intensely visualised by the subject. If the pencil is believed to be a burning hot piece of metal, it is imaged and felt as such. The objective condition of the pencil is irrelevant here. It does not matter.

The Dutch and German languages have a special name for this kind of reality, in which this working (practical) quality comes out clearly; worklike (*werkelijkheid* and *Wirklichkeit*). Rationality is only impractical (and useless) theoretical material, as far as the practical emotional mind is concerned. If it works on us, if it has the power to change us, then it is real, and it does not matter if it is rational or not.

Example: a patient visualised his body healing as a technical-mechanical process, much like a carpenter or surgeon would go about working. When I asked him to dream about this, while in a relaxed state, he saw himself as a child in a sailor suit cowering against an enormous evil threatening monster. What was lacking in his neutral technical imagery of chipping away with a chisel at the cancer tissue, was this personal factor of feeling very small and totally helpless against the big monster. This confrontation was accompanied by a sense of fear and despair of not being able to manage the job. The fear had remained unformulated in his mind until then as a vague feeling that had not been put into pictures or words.

This emotional aspect makes it clear what has to be done: the powerful negative image has to change. He must learn to reject that abnormal fear of the mighty cancer and remove the myth from his mind by countering visualisation, reduce the baddie to a more manageable size and enlarge himself to a powerful figure. By systematic practice, he must erase that bad image of a loser situation from his emotional mind until the new positive winning image comes spontaneously.

As long as the original fearful image continued to exist as a guiding image in his emotional mind, all his visualisations of healing would have been a waste of time. Imagery is important in any kind of healing, such as in the psychotherapy of wrong emotional attitudes, and in healing of the body. This kind of imagery has little or nothing to do with the rational mind. It is not intellectual imagination but emotional imagery which has a powerful effect on our organism, because it follows the emotional logic of life. Such emotional images can affect our organism through and through.

Is this not the reason why the image of cancer as a monstrous danger is so effective that it can kill? That a witch doctor's curse can be so powerful in its effect on the hapless victim, especially when the social environment collaborates with his suggestion? It is the emotional meaning of the situation that affects us so deeply, not its rational significance.

Negative emotional images can have such a powerful effect on our organism, therefore positive images have the same magic!

Will telling a child there is no such thing as a monster under its bed satisfy the child, soothe the fear? No effort of reasoning will calm the child because the monster is a real experience that is based on pure emotional logic. Rationality is only an adult invention, and alien in the practical world of the child. Did this frightened child then really see the monster, as he so emphatically claimed?

'You are a little sook', we scoff: 'Monsters don't exist, so you can't possibly have seen it.' No matter how many times the child protests that he really saw the monster, we refuse to believe him. Not that the child is mistaken, but we adults have forgotten our childhood: the child did experience the monster. He will experience the monster even if it has no objective existence.

The logical distinction that adults make between reality and imagination is a rational distinction that the child is simply not yet capable of making, because he still knows absolutely nothing about such grown-up rational logic.

How is it possible that the child really saw the monster? How is it possible that we see it in our own nightmare? We don't walk around in a nightmare denying the reality of this monster because it is also real for us. We are in a state of panic and desperately trying to get away from it. We are not present as waking adults in the dream, but then the child is not a waking adult either, and does not live in the adult reality.

The rational distinction between reality and imagination does not yet exist for the child. The child lives in a different reality, a reality of magic, myth, and mystery, and of a powerfully creative imagination.

This is a practical, workable reality for our emotional mind, until it becomes distressed. Then this practical emotional mind becomes disorganised and no longer practical, which means that it is no longer useful for maintaining the normal living order. The child may experience monsters that can severely frighten it in a reality that has now become impractical and unfamiliar under the disorganising influence of its distress.

We must not think that the world of myth and magic is merely a useless fairy tale world of the child and of the childlike imagination of the adult. It is a practical way of looking at an uncertain reality, that can ease the emotional mind in its many moments of doubt and apprehension. This was the important conclusion of Ernst Cassirer, one of the profound thinkers of our century, after a comprehensive study of the subject (E. Cassirer, *Philosophy of symbolic forms, volume three*).

It explains the capricious behaviour of an unpredictable world in practical terms. It tells us about the deities that decide our fate and this is very important, it gives us the opportunity to do something concrete about this fate. We can influence fate by actively involving ourselves with it. We can bring offerings to ensure goodwill, for example. We are never helpless bystanders here, we participate in our fate.

A rational explanation of reality takes all that away from us; it makes us stand aloof from it, so that we are now reduced to being helpless spectators of the show, without any effective input. This situation is fine for a computer, but for humans, the feeling of helplessness is an emotional illness.

The classical explanation of this unpredictable world has been shown to be wrong; the more modern quantum physics states that we are inevitably involved in the creation of our own sensory world. In short: the world is there because we are here.

For the child there is originally no difference between seeing and imagining the world. This means that there is originally no difference between the reality that we experience, and the realm that we imagine. This is why the technique of visualisation is effective in bringing about bodily changes.

For this to be effective, we must shift away from our ordinary adult waking state, and switch off the doubting adult rational mind that has caused the separation and that will maintain it for as long as we are awake.

The child can have great influence over its body, but does not know how to use it. Adults can use it, but lack the original closeness between mind and body of the child. A child has only to imagine itself being sick, to vomit immediately. That is why we must learn to lose our rational adult state if we want to visualise effectively.

Inactivation of the rational mind can be done by shifting into an altered state of consciousness. This happens normally when we fall asleep, when we daydream, when our emotions run high, and when we are tired or otherwise unwell. It also takes a back seat when the sobering light of day disappears. When it gets dark, we may feel romantic or fearful, depending on the current direction of our intensified creative imagination.

This altered state can also be brought about by hypnosis, by self-relaxation or through intense emotions. The rational mind is also inactivated in the dream, but here we do not have much control over the changing nature of the visual images, and the direction that they take.

The extraordinary capacity of the wholeheartedly visualising emotional mind to produce marked bodily changes has been well documented; the bleeding hands and the crown of thorns pattern of bleeding on the forehead in religious fervour, are examples of the effect of visualisation during intense concentration. Second degree burns have been produced by hypnotic suggestion, and the clearing of various skin disorders has been brought about with the same method. The story of hypnosis is replete with such examples.

All these effects are produced by creative visualisation of a single image in total, prolonged, and intense concentration. Another ingredient is, of course, faith: in God or, for our purposes, preferably in ourselves: faith in our ability to be effective in our own defence and healing. Faith concentrates our emotional mind, and makes it effective.

However we visualise, we have to do it in full concentration, and with total abandon. Halfhearted attempts at visualisation are not very effective, and if wholeheartedness does not come spontaneously, then we only need to practise it in a learning process.

The child will eventually learn to make the adult distinction between practical sensory experience and idle imagination, but even as an adult it will quite often return involuntarily to this original state: in dreaming or under the intoxicating and hypnotising influence of strong emotions.

Professor Pierre Janet, an eminent French psychiatrist at the turn of the century, wrote of a patient who was plagued by fearful images, and who managed (supported by Janet) to overcome them by turning the evil person of her imagery into a clown. When this visualised change was successful, her fears disappeared. Reasoning with her would have been useless and out of place.

That is a good example of making an effective use of positive emotional logic to combat wrong emotional logic. Instead of scolding a fearful child in the mistaken belief that we are teaching her rational logic, it is much more effective to use magic to remove the monster from the room. Many intuitive mothers practise it with good effect. While in such a fearful state, it is not the right time to teach the child rational logic anyway. Only a calm child can become open to reason.

Rational logic is the logic of our human intellect when we are merely idling, when we are not doing anything urgent or new that requires the attention of our practical emotional mind. If we wish to teach it to the child, then we should wait for the right time, when the child is in the right frame of mind; at rest, and emotionally settled.

Rational logic is powerless against emotional logic; when they clash, it is always the stronger and older emotional logic that is the winner. The logic of our emotional mind is in the driver's seat, after all.

A smoker complains that he cannot stop smoking in spite of all rational advice: 'You will ruin your arteries and lungs if you don't stop. Every puff of a cigarette now is a lost breath later. Every cigarette will cost you some functioning lung tissue.' His answer: 'I know all that doc, I just can't help it.'

A distressed emotional mind is in the driver's seat and tells the smoker to continue to smoke, not to take any notice of any advice given by anybody's rational mind. Our emotional mind is normally practical (life-promoting), but it becomes abnormal and erratic in its instructions during stress, because stress disorganises it.

Emotional instructions, after all, are directions according to emotional logic. The practical emotional mind, as we said, is in the driver's seat; the rational mind is merely a commenting passenger in our organism. The emotional mind was born for the driver's seat, and was already there at birth. It only had to learn the technique of practical driving in the first few years.

We are born as emotional creatures, but we have to develop a rational mind from the age of two and a half. Our emotional mind is the first-born, and it is always the older and more powerful in its effect on the body.

As long as it is not stressed, our guiding emotional mind can only issue practical, effective life-sustaining, instructions.

During stress our emotional mind becomes disorganised, and begins to give out wrong commands that can play havoc with the practical order of the body.

A rational approach to healing does not work unless you stick to medication and other physical therapies that can over-ride your emotional mind. If you wish to use your mind to assist in healing, use your emotional mind, and use the same strategies and logic that it uses. A doctor visualised a precise surgical operation on his cancer, but was surprised to dream of his cancer as a terrifying black-gowned figure about to embrace him fatally, as he recoiled from it in panic.

Emotional logic is a very strange logic when we view it from a rational point of view, yet children accept it as natural, as do we adults in our dreams and fantasies. This is the logic of myths, legends, and fairy tales: stories that are rationally impossible because they go against the grain of our invented rational logic.

Our emotional mind has been called a mythopoeic mind, a practical myth-creating mind which is an effective tool for dealing with an uncertain reality. These myths and fairy tales are not created for nothing. They have a practical function because they help us cope with a capricious reality that is not at all rational. Rational explanations are not for immediate coping. They are theories: ideas that have no immediate practical benefit for an organism that must act quickly to survive.

The rational mind uses abstract theoretical concepts such as numbers, chance, statistical probability and averages, to try to make rational sense of a chaotic reality in which nothing is certain until the very moment that it happens. It tries to understand reality in terms of invented theoretical concepts.

The emotional mind, on the other hand, prefers to work with practical beliefs that will help it to manage, to cope with that capricious reality. Our rational understanding is not necessary for practical coping with life.

Our emotional mind is the mind that we must rely on in visualisation. We relax our body first; we immobilise it to free our mind from its practical task of guiding the body in its action. By turning our interested attention away from the outside world, we unhitch our emotional mind from its active duties. We close our eyes to that world, we sit or lie totally still so that we don't feel around for it. We can now turn our attention to our body, and use our liberated emotional mind for the purpose of visualising our recovery and well-being.

STRUCTURE AND CHANGE

One great hindrance to effective self-assistance in healing is that the rational mind cannot believe in the possibility of the mind changing the body. This disbelief has nothing to do with reality; it is an illusion that has been created by a mechanistic set of mind.

In this outdated way of understanding, the mind is thought to be of immaterial substance. Once we define it in this way, how can it ever connect with the body? Without going into the problem any deeper, let me just say that the mind is the free and changeable part of our organism, and the body is the steady, and less changing part. We call this fixed part an anatomical structure, and we label the free part as a mind.

Our rational mind has been educated wrongly in matters of life (medicine, biology). The body was studied first as a structure (anatomy) and only later as a function (physiology). We began studying a mechanistic biology before psychology. Medicine had its priorities wrong because it studied the part before it considered the whole.

The emotional mind is the function of the total organism, and is its variable part, the easily changeable part. The body is the sum of our more fixed routines.

Even so, this does not mean that they cannot be changed only that it takes longer to change a body routine than to change our mind. Without going into this too much, let me just ask you to see your body as a routine that the mind uses for its habitual tasks.

A scary thought sets our heart pounding and we experience the emotion of fear. A scary thought is an emotional thought, and our nervous system cannot detect the difference between reality and imagination. It receives this information, and translates it into the appropriate code for the support and action systems that must deal with this danger. Our organism is mobilised, primed for action. The palpitations come with an urge to go into action. If there is no actual danger, the uproar settles down after a while.

A neutral thought, coming from our rational mind, could never activate us like this because it is only our emotional mind that sits in the driver's seat behind the body controls. If our stressed emotional mind (which is now an over-emotional and over-sensitive mind) dreams up a fearful thought, it can't tell that this is imagination, and not the practical reality. The alarm of danger is passed on to the nervous system.

If we can't get rid of the scary thought, then we become jumpy and nervous all the time, and it shows in our attitude and our continuing palpitations. If we stay in this aroused state too long, the pattern may become chronic: fixed in actual biochemical changes in the involved organ systems.

This happens all the time in normal adaptations. For example, if we use our muscles more, those that are exercised will grow in size. Muscles not in regular use shrink. Athletes develop a slower pulse rate. Nervous persons develop a raised pulse rate while regularly angry people may get ulcers, hypertension or other problems. The constant suppression of anger is fixed in a number of more serious psychosomatic illnesses. Our constitution plays an important role in this. The constitution is best thought of as an inborn talent for acquiring or resisting the creation of problems or of positive achievements.

This fixing in stable patterns (chronification) of regularly occurring change is not surprising, because this is nature's rule for an efficient biological economy: whatever must last will be fixed in some bodily change.

If we must water our garden regularly, for example, it would be more efficient to arrange a hose to run from the tap to the garden, than having to run back and forth with water held in our two cupped hands.

The body is not a thing, it is a movement that is so slowed down, that we see it as a structure, because this is practical for all organismic activity. This body form acts as a funnel for proper action, and goes a long way towards making sure that our organism stays in the direction of health.

If our body has strayed from the narrow path of health, we only have to re-orientate it, nudge it back in the proper direction. And this is precisely what can be done in visualisation.

We can try to change the wrong direction by physical methods. We can use medicines or surgery to force our organism to steer itself back onto the right track. But we can also use the emotional mind for the purpose, because this mind is, after all, the body's natural steering wheel.

Dr Georg Groddeck, a famous German physician and the father of psychosomatic medicine (and a friend of Freud), said that a doctor's healing job is to get the natural biological organisation of the body going, to activate this biocomputer, and steer it in the direction of healing and well-being. He did not call it a biocomputer, but he might have, if he had lived long enough. Instead, he called it the It (*das Es*).

Freud took that over as a better name for the unconscious, but Groddeck's 'It' went much deeper. What this It is, he said, I can't tell you: I only use it as a working image. But I can tell you what it does! It makes sick, and It heals. Who heals the wound? he asked. It is certainly not the doctor. He merely stitches it up; not the patient herself either, but that complicated organisation that runs all living functions, from our heartbeat to healing and defence. Something heals, and that something, said Groddeck, that X, that unknown entity, I call the It. The doctor treats, the patient helps, but It does the real work: It does the healing.

Surgical and oncological treatment intervenes, but it takes more than that to heal: It, the *vis medicatrix naturae*, must be invoked to de-stress, activate, and re-direct the organism from its wrong course. And this can be done through relaxation and visualisation.

I repeat: don't be fussed if your visualisation runs counter to all rational logic. You are not involved in any classical physical experiment. You are working on a reality that runs according to an emotional logic.

Chapter Seventeen

WORKING WITH MODELS

WORKING HYPOTHESIS

When we decide to work on a particular project, we always have natural expectations about the way in which it should come out. Should we decide to build a house, for example, we fully expect to succeed and that the house will be more or less as we designed it. If we didn't have this expectation, there would simply be no point in building it.

Sometimes we must express the expectation deliberately and explicitly: we think out a working model of how the progress and outcome of the project are going to be; thus we define a working hypothesis. This is no more than a theory that guides our work in the near future, a design for this future to guide our efforts.

We may not even be aware that we are using a working model. We decide to get up from our chair with the intention of going to the letterbox to collect our mail. The working model that we unconsciously adopt here, is that we shall succeed in doing just that. We get out of bed in the morning with the silent expectation that the world is not going to collapse, and that we shall live through a normal day. Otherwise, why should we bother to get up?

Everything we do is based on some working model of succeeding. If we catch a cold, we expect, we even take it for granted, that we shall get better. This is our biological right; we all have a powerful regulation system that allows us to recover from such a disturbance of our organism.

At times, however, doubt may creep in. Will we get over this complication? What if we don't, or what if we should get worse? We are now no longer taking our earlier working model for granted. We bring up an alternative, a different possible design for our future.

Only in two situations do we ask such questions:

 (i) When we want to express reasonable doubts;

 (ii) When we are not really asking, but complaining; this will happen when we are down in the dumps, so that we are merely giving voice to the thoroughly disheartened and miserable way we feel.

Let us understand clearly that such questions about the future exist only in our mind; we are concerned about our future, and we express this concern, but such concern is no prediction of the actual future. It is too easy to lose sight of this difference, and to start believing in these doubts, as if they were reality rather than merely questions in our mind. Motivated by our misery, we may believe that we are finished, and use this as a working model, unless we learn to manage our emotional mind better.

Some important rules in the management of our emotional states are given below. We use these to avoid adopting a negative working model that may harm us.

(a) Whenever we are in the grip of abnormal emotions (such as anxiety, anger or depression) our emotional mind is no longer a reliable guide to reality. We can now no longer take it for granted that what we may think and believe about the world is correct. In stress, our practical emotional mind leaves us in the lurch, and it can now only misguide us while our rational mind is hard to find.

(b) We deal with this by remembering: 'I refuse to believe in whatever my misguiding emotional mind may tell me about the world. I shall look at the situation again when I have calmed down, and only then make any decisions that have to be made.'

This is made much easier by relaxing at the same time. Wait and relax for a more useful second look.

(c) 'What if' complaints have nothing to do with the future. 'What if' as a lament only points to a negative state of mind, and it is no more than a complaint of emotional discomfort.

(d) If they are not useful questions, reject them as firmly as you can, and use all the emotional support that you can get to achieve this. Use this time more profitably, because you are only

indulging in negative visualisation, while you should be busy with
doing the opposite, with positive visualisation.

WHICH WORKING MODEL?

We must now make a choice; we either work to get better or we
let our health slide by default. We must make a decision. Which
of the two working models for a future do we wish to adopt?
Make your selection:

(i) *I am going to fight and recover fully,* or:

(ii) *I give up without even trying.*

If we select the first option we must rehearse it in order to put
it into effect. The second option does not need deliberate
rehearsing: that is already done by the negative state of mind and
is motivated by wrong emotions.

You have no other choice. If you do not deliberately adopt the
positive working hypothesis then you automatically select the
negative one. That is the expectation of failing to recover from
the illness. Fence-sitting also means adopting the negative
working model.

The working model becomes a guideline for the emotional
mind that now begins its work towards the future, for better or
worse. Our future cannot happen without input from us; we have
a say, because we cannot help taking part.

In the proverbial dentist's chair, for example, we begin to brace
automatically against possible pain. This bracing makes us feel
twice as much pain, because we adopt the working model that it
is going to hurt. Tensing up increases our sensitivity to pain. If we
have a confident expectation that we are not going to be
bothered by pain, we shall feel less (if any) pain.

Good hypnotic subjects have an easily accepting (suggestible)
mind, that is capable of instantly and strongly believing in a
suggestion.

'It does not hurt!' The suggestion is strongly visualised and
accepted as a certainty, and this happens quite spontaneously.
And here is the magic: it does not hurt.

The doubting personality can't seem to accept the suggestion,
and worries at it: Let me check that . . . What if . . . Yes but . . . We
can understand that if one says: 'That's all very well that it is not
going to hurt, but what if it does?' This means that it is probably

going to hurt, because the suggestion is being rejected and prevented from working. This personality cannot help bringing up the alternative possibility. Suggest black and instantly the doubt comes; what if it should be white. This kind of fence-sitting represents an inability to go one way or the other. The vacillation is also known as ambivalence, an inability to commit oneself, based on a sense of insecurity.

The doubter personality keeps wavering between two options. One moment it wants to believe in one, but in the next is afraid that it is the other. The doubter personality must now deliberately rehearse the positive working model in order to commit her/himself to it. In other words, this favourable outcome must be trained-in like an athletic performance. Such practice will overcome the wavering, and allow the model to ripen and gradually sink in. If we deliberately relax and rehearse the hypothesis: 'When I am relaxed, I shall suffer little pain', we commit ourselves to feeling little pain, and we shall feel little pain.

USING THE EMOTIONAL MIND

Animals and humans are born for action, as I have said. They have been designed and built for it. To make action more effective, all living beings which can move around need a guiding system to choose the most effective form of action for the current situation.

Lower animals have a primitive guiding system that is composed of instincts. They are relatively rigid commands for direct action that have a powerful compelling quality, and that must be obeyed without hesitation. Such instincts are not sufficiently adaptable for dealing with more complicated situations, though. The primitive guiding system is an instinctive mind.

In higher animals and human beings, nature has invented a new version of this guiding system. It is much more flexible and adaptable to rapidly changing circumstances. It is an emotional mind that is like a newer version of the existing instinct program. Not for nothing do feelings come and go. They are perfectly adapted to the changing world in which situations also come and go.

The newer guiding system (compare it to an upgraded software program) has taken over from our instinctive mind because it is just as fast but more flexible. The new version is a more efficient guiding system for behaviour. It allows for errors, and can bring alternative strategies into action. Instincts may be amazingly precise, but there is no room for error in the instinct-guided system.

This function of allowing for errors is a sign of improvement that can also be found in the history of computers. The early line-editors were rigid and would crash after a mistake. Newer versions have error-handling functions, that make them more flexible and useful, more user-friendly. Emotions are more user-friendly than the more rigid instincts.

Both the instinctive and emotional minds are practical guiding systems that can find the most effective form of action in most situations.

Guidance means: the planning of the most efficient action to be taken in a particular situation. In other words: selecting the most practical working model and putting it to work. All this is done by means of feelings (all kinds of sensations and emotions). Feeling good about the future means our emotional mind has adopted a positive working model, even if we don't know it. Feeling bad about the future implies that it has chosen a negative working model.

We can influence our emotional mind to produce a positive working model through the use of relaxation and visualisation. We can set our emotional mind on a positive course.

Every move that we make in life is based on a working model of the immediate future. We can never know what this future looks like. It is never certain in advance. Small causes can have enormous effects. Our own input, tiny as it may seem, can change the future considerably as it develops towards becoming the present.

We can only guess about this future. One person's guess is as good as the next. When some doctor gives an opinion about the outcome of a disorder, this is no more than an educated guess, based on statistical averages. The doctor is therefore not talking about your future but of that of the patient public. Nobody can predict your individual future because there is no statistical average for one person.

If someone says to you: you might as well give me your Tatts ticket, because the statistical average of winning is against you, would you be so foolish as to part with it? No. Who knows, you might win. The gods of chaos don't deal with statistical averages. Their system of mathematics is much too complicated for us to understand. We can only try to understand chaos with our own invented working models.

Since the beginning of humankind, we have been using myths and other beliefs to understand uncertain reality. Modern scientists use the method of statistics and mathematics to understand unpredictable reality. Other people still use the older, practical method of the emotional mind; they work with beliefs. In either case, everyone is working with models about the nature of reality and about the future, and such working models are our own creations.

Before the seventeenth century, people said that gods decided the future. After the scientific revolution in that century an impersonal and scientific god called chance took their place. This was the predictable god of numbers and of numerical probabilities. We were not much better off.

Now physicists speak about a totally unpredictable chaos that decides the future, and reality begins to look very strange to the baffled rational mind trying to make it fit into a rational system. All this means: our reality, and the future that belongs to it, is uncertain and unpredictable, and always will be.

The doctor should only state: 'I can tell you the averages, Mr TCP, but I can't tell what will happen in your particular case. That is anybody's guess, and you will have to make up your own mind about that.'

Refuse to accept anything else, particularly if it sounds like bone-pointing. Make all the legal, financial, and other arrangements that are necessary because of the risk involved to relieve yourself of that responsibility. If the family wants quality time with you, by all means give it to them, provided it does not have the effect of bone-pointing, and without letting go of the positive working model.

Having attended to all that, now you can concentrate on getting over the cancerous infection.

Bone-pointing statements such as: 'You have six months, with luck ten months' and 'You won't see Christmas, I'm afraid', are guesses. They apply to the average person and not to you. Your reply should be similar to the reply that the patient gave her surgeon: 'You may know your statistics, but you don't know me.'

We cannot know the future. We base our life, and all our projects on one or other working model of the future. We only adopt a self-defeating working model when, in our state of total demoralisation, we have lost all hope.

In this condition, there is no positive working model because we can't see any future for ourselves. But this lack of a future has nothing to do with biology. It is our emotional state of mind that closes off the future. We have a biological right to recover from any illness. To say that something is hopeless is either to pretend to see into a totally unpredictable future, or it is just a complaint about feeling miserable. In either case, it has no bearing on your future. If you feel that your case is hopeless, that is only your private opinion. Just don't practise it constantly.

Expect to recover; that is your biological right. Use that as a working model for a reality in which anything may happen, and use it whether you suffer from an infection with bacteria, cancer cells, parasites, or viruses. Having made all necessary practical arrangements, we should now leave all doubts behind and concentrate on the hypothesis that we are going to heal. We take this as our working model for the future, and begin our rehearsal for recovery.

Take a closer look at the idea of working models of the future and what they can do for us. Remember: you are not fooling yourself. You are deliberately adopting this model for rehearsal. It allows you to take charge, to fight for your health, rather than sinking into becoming a passive and despairing patient, a TCP.

Chapter Eighteen

TWO WORKING MODELS

There are only two possible working models of the future that we can use regarding the cancer infection, and the situation is this: if it is not one then it is the other. It is either: I get well or: I don't get well (I remain chronically sick or I die). It is important that we realise this, if we wish to get rid of the voodoo. Let us look at these two possibilities.

I get well. This means that we adopt an active attitude towards the illness: 'I am going to get well and I am going to work on it myself. I am going to take charge of this situation because I myself must deal with this. I am in the driver's seat and from here, I delegate responsibility to my assistants whoever they may be.'

'If I employ an oncologist to look after the biological side of cancer, I shall trust her (him) with that job, and I am not going to worry myself sick from day to day about test results. I will (if I can manage this) let the oncologist worry about it, because that is her (his) specialty and responsibility.

'I myself will be too busy with: getting rid of the voodoo, and getting myself in top condition for the fight against the biological cancer, as much as I can. I have a full-time job on my hands. I have to become fighting fit, with good morale: a trained soldier at the front. Healing and surviving is my responsibility. Whatever treatment I get from my medical assistants, I try to use to my own benefit. If I feel pain or experience discomfort I try, as much as I can, to cope with it.'

Don't only think of what the discomfort of radio/ chemotherapy (if any) means for the cancer cells, but concentrate wholly on that. Shift the focus of your pain and discomfort from your own body to the cancer, if you can, and do it whenever you can relax enough to concentrate.

It is also helpful to the oncologist that you have the same positive attitude you expect from her or him. Attitudes and the emotions behind them are highly infectious. If you infect the oncologist with a negative attitude, she or he will be affected by it. Nobody is so resistant that she or he cannot be infected with emotions.

We have infections of the mind (with wrong emotions) as well as those of the body with micro-organisms and cancer, and we have self-protective systems of the emotional mind as well as those of the body.

Some personalities have highly resistant emotional minds; they pick on everything you say, question it, turn it around and around in their mind, find fault with it, and can usually only accept a little bit of it at best.

They don't do this deliberately because they couldn't accept a suggestion easily, even if they wanted to. They seem to have a finicky mental digestive system. This would sound fine if it were not for the fact that they question and doubt themselves all the time also.

At the other extreme, we see personalities who accept every suggestion too easily; they are easily infected with someone else's emotions and suggestions, and they tend to pass it on. Mr TCP belongs to this group. The weakness in the defensive system seems to lie not only in the bodily resistance but also in that of the mind. Mr TCP gets clinical cancer and picks up the voodoo curse as well. Fortunately, an alternative working model can be adopted just as easily.

I don't get well. This is the working model that Mr TCP uses. He is demoralised from the beginning by accepting the voodoo. In certain people this negative working theory becomes a certainty from the start. It is not even a working model any more, it is a conviction so that their minds have locked over it, like a delusion.

This wrong working model of the future is a faulty expectation that can be changed. The voodoo can be lifted. Mr TCP is then free to adopt the better working hypothesis. He throws off his demoralised state and usually feels and looks almost instantly more healthy.

If I say: 'I can't believe that I can recover from cancer or any other infection', such a statement only means that I have a negative belief, the belief of not being able to recover. This is no more than a poor working model of the future which I believe in. This is merely a belief, and not a prediction of the future. It exists only in the emotional mind, not in reality itself. It is a wrong belief that is entertained in the emotional mind, a demon, an emotional virus that preys on the mind, but does not exist in concrete reality.

The choice of this negative working model does not have to be deliberate. If you don't accept the positive working model, then you accept the negative model by default, automatically. With such a working model, what else can one do but give up? And this is exactly what Mr TCP does. He is demoralised; he feels helpless, hopeless, is in total despair, he is resigned to dying soon. He is giving up without a fight, by abandoning himself totally to the abnormal hypnotic suggestion that he is doomed, that he must die. He is in a state of emotional failure.

Mr TCP is well and truly caught in an emotional voodoo trap. His organism is in a state of failure, of disorganisation, so that even its life-support regulating systems are no longer working properly. One typical result of this is that his digestion packs up; he loses his appetite, and loses weight. His defence and healing systems have shut down, because he has dropped his bundle. Things are now badly wrong, because the disordered regulating system can no longer take care of what is going on.

His entire internal self-servicing system is in disrepair; it is itself now in a state of disorganisation, so Mr TCP is on an unnecessary downward slide. His system is dysfunctional. It can no longer recognise the invasion, and can no longer defend and maintain his organism.

Mr TCP allows his medical and social environment to continue their unknowing bone-pointing behaviour towards him, without resistance, without bothering to fight: he is apathetic. The typical cancer patient syndrome is a demoralisation syndrome. Mr TCP has given up living and is resigned to dying. This is an abnormal resignation that is associated with deep apathy; an illness of the emotional mind that can occur in any serious entrapment. There is no future in this working model. This is meant both literally and as a figure of speech. This working model does not include a future, and there is no benefit in adopting it. This is only a wrong belief. It says absolutely nothing about the future, because nobody can foretell the future. There is no need to die from such a wrong belief, because you have an alternative. Choose the better one. What can you lose? This one has an open future and represents hope.

Some doctors believe that one should accept the cancer gracefully, and enjoy the days left in intimate contact with family and friends. They advise not to waste time with relaxation or meditation or other such fringe pastimes. This is usually a specialist view from an ivory tower, and only rarely the front-line experience of a perceptive general practitioner. Who on earth can enjoy today, knowing that tomorrow brings death? We suspect that there is something wrong with the person who stoically accepts a death sentence. Freud, who in his old age suffered stoically from a jaw cancer, was one of these, but he was elderly, and perhaps felt that he had a reputation to maintain.

Very few people, if any, could accept a death sentence with grace and equanimity, or with a rational attitude and without emotional turmoil. There is more likely to be a denial of life behind this façade, a strong motive for rejecting a biological existence.

Ask any person in panic or despair if she or he can enjoy the day. Ask a deeply worried person to enjoy herself, and she will simply answer: 'I can't, I feel too anxious for that, too much on edge and apprehensive, too restless.'

Three other points should be clarified for such doctors, and for other people with similar attitudes:

(a) The indifference of scientific medicine to the negative effects of emotions in healing, wrote Professor Jerome Frank, may account for many treatment failures, and also drives people to look for alternative forms of healing. He quotes B. Inglis as saying that people do that not because they are naive or stupid, but because they seek the support there that they cannot find in traditional medical doctors who are usually too busy with techniques of drug treatment to bother about emotional support (page 47).

When cancer patients go to fringe practitioners, we only have ourselves to blame. It is because we fall short in this important area of emotional support.

(b) To call relaxation and visualisation 'alternative' medicine would upset more than half the psychotherapists of Europe and the United States if they were to take it seriously. Autogenic training, for example, with or without the use of visualisation, is a well established and highly respected and effective psychotherapeutic technique.

Psychotherapy with the cancer patient is not an alternative form of therapy of the biological cancer, and some oncologists would do well to be more open to the need for psychological support of their patients, particularly the TCPs.

The emotional load that such patients carry is too heavy, and causes too much suffering, to be ignored. The cancer patient is not a biological mechanism, but first and foremost a highly sensitive human being, and a psychosomatic unit.

(c) Only very elderly people can have a calm attitude towards death. They may feel that they have had a full life and that it is all right that the end is coming because they feel ready for it. There is more to this however. The older we become, the less we seem to become involved with emotional issues that were so important earlier in life.

This is a natural phenomenon that has practical value: older persons say that they are too old to worry too much about such things. It is as if Mother Nature protects them from excessive suffering.

Chapter Nineteen

REQUIREMENTS FOR HEALING

Healing requires an appropriate state of mind. It does not matter whether we are trying to heal from a wound, cancer, a broken leg, or from pneumonia: the principles remain the same. Healing has a biological side and a psychological side:

Biologically, healing requires the wound to be clean of infection, and the invaders removed. The wound must then still heal from the damage.

Psychologically, healing requires a healing atmosphere for the organism. Our emotional mind is intimately involved with the creation of this vital healing atmosphere. We need to call up this special atmosphere before proper biological healing can take place, in the same way that digestion is most efficient in a dining atmosphere. A properly prepared stomach, with its digestive juices flowing and digestive movements activated by the promise of good eating, welcomes the food when it arrives.

Resting the body is needed to prevent movement from aggravating the condition and to avoid pain. It is equally necessary to relax the emotional mind away from activity and stress, so that healing can begin. We must prepare our organism for healing by creating the right atmosphere for it.

We know that infected wounds don't heal, and that stress prevents proper wound healing. We are so used to ignoring the role of the mind in the healing of minor infections and wounds that we often forget to take into account the emotional mind of the person with more serious problems. Even an animal looks for an appropriate shelter to heal: a place of rest for the body and for its emotional mind. It is a safe place, a stress-free zone in which the body is secure, so that the mind can then become free from the needs of action and devote itself to healing.

Ignoring the role of the mind in healing is a typical outcome of our preoccupation with technical advances in medicine. Doctors put more faith in medication and surgery than in the *vis medicatrix naturae*, which they take for granted. It is usually only when our medical technique fails that we appeal to the healing powers of nature. We do only as a last resort what we should be doing from the start.

If we wish to use our emotional mind for effective healing, we should unharness it from action and bind it to healing. That requires proper preparation. By creating the right conditions we can have access to a reserve healing capacity.

The state of the emotional mind is important in the matter of healing in another respect too. This emotional mind, as we said, is in the driver's seat of the organism. If it is disorganised in stress then all its instructions to the body will be equally disorganised. In addition to the dysfunctional emotional mind, we have now also a dysfunctional body whose functions are no longer practical. These functions are now no longer appropriate and effective, they are no longer working normally for our health. A stressed emotional mind is not the right instrument for healing.

We only have to glance at the list of possible stress symptoms to realise how severe this disorganisation of the workings of the body can be. There is a large assortment of such symptoms and signs of stress: headaches, dizziness, ringing in the ears, tired and sore eyes, no appetite, nausea, stomach pains and knots, indigestion, diarrhoea, bowel cramps, constipation, bladder frequency, pains in the chest, palpitations, wheezing, coughing, shortness of breath, itchy skin, rashes, aches and pains, pains in neck and back, anxiety, panic, depression, loss of enjoyment, irritability, weariness, general weakness, anger, insomnia, cold sweats, hot and cold shivers, sexual dysfunctions, and many more.

What do we notice when we look at that list? Not one of these symptoms is in any way useful for the organism. These experiences are no longer practical sensations and emotions. A rapid pulse rate is normal during fear, because fear is a practical emotion that turns the organism into an effective running machine in times of actual danger.

As we run from danger, we also heat up and perspire. This is due to an effective heat exchange. It allows excessive body heat during action to evaporate so that it prevents the body from overheating. Palpitations and sweating when running, are therefore useful effects of regulation. Our digestive system closes down when we become busy because we have no time for feeding and excreting. This shut-down produces the typical dry mouth in tension, and the stopping of the bowel movements during activity.

But when we have palpitations while just sitting in a state of anxiety where is the benefit of that? Why should we have a pounding pulse, and perspire so profusely, when we are not even exerting ourselves? In anxiety we usually experience a knot in the stomach from an excessive stomach spasm, we may vomit, and feel bowel urgency, have diarrhoea or constipation, we feel hot and cold at the same time: all useless signs and symptoms of stress. Idiomatic expressions are to the point here: we say that we are 'scared shitless', or that it 'scares the shit out of us'. These do not belong to normal fear, but to anxiety, to stress, to a dysfunctional organism.

Such anxiety symptoms can only mean that our organism is in a state of disorganisation. These symptoms are the expression of that condition of dysfunction.

Fear is a purposeful emotion that organises us for appropriate action, while anxiety paralyses us. It makes us useless, dysfunctional. Anxiety is part of stress: it is part of the disorganisation that stress produces. Anxiety, like anger, is always an abnormal feeling, no matter how much romantic existentialist writers try to glorify it.

This disorganisation will affect the internal servicing system so that it may interfere with the proper regulation of defence and healing, for example. Stressed people heal badly, and they take longer than usual to recover even from common infections. If this stress-induced condition of disorganisation is severe enough, it will seriously compromise our self-protective and self-supportive internal functions. That is why healing must take place in a stress-free zone.

Healing also requires that our mind is free from stress and also free from any preoccupation with our everyday affairs: free from anything that requires bodily activity. Why is this?

Our organism is by nature action-orientated; in this sense, we are like a car that has been designed for driving. Driving is its natural purpose. But this wears it out, so it requires frequent servicing, regular repair and maintenance work by competent mechanics.

Our emotional mind is an action-prone guiding system; it is a pilot that is geared to practical activity. It is naturally focused on effective action. This mind selects the most efficient form of action for the current situation, and instructs the body to perform that. This coded instruction is what we call a feeling (sensation or emotion). We have to undo this action-orientation when we wish to undergo internal servicing. We must free our mind from all thoughts to action, from its natural attraction to the world of sights and sounds and textures.

When we rest our body but don't rest our emotional mind from its preoccupation with action, all we get is a grease and oil change. For a major service, we must first switch over the emotional mind from its natural orientation to action to that of healing. We should do this in the same routine way in which we stop working, wash our hands, and come to the table to eat. We shift into a different mode. The shift into relaxation does not come as naturally as going into action. We must relax to free our emotional mind from its action-gearing. We must also learn to relax. We have no ready-made instincts for it.

We have an action system plus an internal servicing system, and we need to be at rest while we recuperate in the same way a car has to be standing quite still, with the engine off, before the mechanics will come out to work on it. Our action system is an ergotropic (energy-using) system, whereas our system for repair and maintenance is a trophotropic (self-servicing) system. This trophotropic system is a recovery or recuperation system, and it is only switched on while we rest our action system.

Healing must take place in a stress-free and action-free zone. Our practical-emotional mind must shift into the recovery mode in which it has to let go of all thoughts of action, and gear itself to instructing the body to heal. To achieve this, as we shall see, we must relax the body. We must immobilise it so the emotional mind can be uncoupled from its natural function of action-guidance. It is now free to be used for other purposes, such as healing.

This instinctive devotion to healing happens spontaneously and naturally in children and animals. In them the more primitive instinctive mind guides the healing system. Dogs instinctively search for a dry, warm, quiet, safe, and darkened place when they are hurt or sick. They look for a shelter, a stress-free and safe atmosphere in which they can devote their organism to healing.

The spontaneous switch to the healing mode can no longer be guaranteed in adults who rest with the body, but find it difficult to rest the busy emotional mind. This mind can only be used to heal when it has been released beforehand. It is the relaxed and quietened mind, the eased mind that has been freed from all preoccupation with doing, that is prepared for recuperation.

Only then can it attend to healing, and spontaneously devote itself to defence and to repair and maintenance work for health. This devotion is a concentration on healing, the alternative to concentrating on the world of action. When relaxed, even a thought of healing spurs it on. An image of healing is even better, and the feeling of healing is best.

Action, and healing and defence, are mutually exclusive systems. If the engine is running, the mechanics will not work on the car. They want the engine switched off and cooled before they will start servicing the car. The short formula is: if action is on, then healing is off, and vice versa.

Furthermore, we must nudge the freed emotional mind in the direction of healing in case it has lost this spontaneous and natural turn. How? By visualising that direction. This is a learning process: visualisation must be rehearsed during relaxation to be effective.

It is performance training. It has nothing at all to do with mysticism; it is the serious training of the body in becoming more competent in self-protection.

Chapter Twenty

GENERAL PRINCIPLES OF HEALING

When an organism is resting from its activities, it is being serviced while it waits and rests. After the rest it feels fit again, because it has been made ready for more action. It has been primed for more work. This process of internal servicing, or priming, is also known as recuperation.

Recuperation means bringing the previously active, but now tired, system back to that normal and orderly practical state which we call good health or well-being. It is basically a routine and regular internal servicing of the working system. We undergo a major internal service while we rest, if we can rest both body and mind.

When an organism has been hurt or sick, then the process that repairs it, and brings it back to its normal fit state, is activated. This is healing and, like recuperation, it begins as soon as we switch off our action system, but not before. Whether it is our arm or leg, or our whole organism, we must rest it when it is sick or injured, if we want it to heal. Healing means becoming whole again, restoring the damaged organism to its original condition of practical well-being. This healing process involves:

(i) restoration (curing) of any local disorder;

(ii) restoration (healing) of the whole organism.

In both recuperation and healing, the servicing function will always affect our complete organism, no matter how trivial the disturbance (tiredness or disorder) may be. A slight cold will affect the entire organism, even if it does not produce clinical signs and symptoms. A local disorder is an abstract concept and not a biological reality because the organism always responds as one unit. A boil on the leg is a matter of concern for the whole organism. The leg is connected to the rest of the organism, is part of the same substance. A leg is a permanent feature of higher organisms only, but an amoeba puts a leg (pseudopod) out and withdraws it into its body when it is no longer needed. Because moving around became a regular need for living, nature fixed this needed movement into a leg for walking (this is another example of the law of biological economy).

The permanent leg remains as much part of the total pool of substance as the temporary leg of the amoeba. The protoplasm (living substance) of the organism forms one whole just as a body of water is one single unit. Stir a pond somewhere, and the effect ripples through the whole pond, even if we cannot follow this into detail.

The total organism is therefore always involved in any healing activity, because the entire organism must be restored to its previously normal (healthy, practical) order.

More generally speaking, any kind of change, good or bad, big or small, that happens to us, will always affect our complete organism in a reorganising or readjusting process, that works to rectify the disturbance. This is regulation: balancing activity that may be directed to outer action-support when the organism is busy, or to internal servicing, when the organism is at rest.

It is not possible to stimulate or move a part of the organism without involving the whole organism. A shift of one foot requires a rearrangement of the balance of the entire organism, not only of the body but also of the mind. A change in attitude also involves a reorganisation of the entire organism, so that both mind and body are affected by it.

It is impossible to move your big toe without involving your whole organism in the movement. To move only your big toe, you must first organise the rest of the body: you must set it so still, that it allows the toe alone to move. The same can be seen in producing the knee reflex; only by bracing the rest of the body can this reflex be allowed to take place seemingly by itself.

It is equally impossible to have a painful ingrowing toenail that does not affect the entire organism to some degree in its discomfort and treatment. The curing of the big toe must involve the entire organism in healing. If the dug-in toenail is infected and painful, who complains? The big toe maybe? Who goes to the doctor for treatment? Does the big toe decide to visit by itself as a statement of independence? Who has to nurse it back to health after surgery? It is you, as the complete organism, who suffers and feels the pain, not your big toe. It is only a small part of you as a total system. It is your job, as its manager, to look after it and keep it well.

For all practical purposes, we may consider the terms mind, organism, you, me, as one and the same entity. Their differences are merely theoretical distinctions, and are important only for academic speculation. Does the big toe employ you to look after it? No, it is you as your emotional mind who uses the toe, who has it available for walking, and who suffers if it is damaged. Now: does your brain employ you to do what has to be done, or do you use your brain to achieve what you want done? The mind contains the body, and it makes use of this body for practical purposes, such as staying alive.

Infected toenail or cancer: the emotional mind, including its personalised part, is always deeply involved with the invasion and the subsequent fight for health.

We shall now concentrate mainly on healing, even though we can never separate it from recuperation and outer regulation.

HEALING

Healing has two main functions:

(a) *Defensive work.* This involves the general defence of the organism: the detection of invasion and its elimination.

(b) *Reparative work.* This is concerned with damage control and repair.

We must understand the following three principles if we want to have a good idea what healing involves:

Principle of biological efficiency and economy. This principle states that whatever change is regularly repeated, will become fixed in a stable pattern. This usually involves becoming fixed in bodily changes. These can be biochemical or even structural changes, but what is fixed is the function. We learn a poem, so that we can recite it when we want. It is not so important how this learnt recital is fixed (as chemical or structural changes), it is more important to realise that the function of reciting the poem is fixed in a stable routine pattern by learning. We see that this is exactly what learning means, forming stable patterns of action.

Whatever this action may be, it must always begin with the emotional mind. Learning to walk, to drive a car, remembering or thinking: all such functions originate in the emotional mind.

If we perform a movement only once, we have made a casual and unique motion, one that can never be exactly repeated in its once-only form. If we try to repeat this movement, we can only reproduce its general pattern, and if we continue to repeat it, we then shave off all the little differences between the individual movements, so that they begin to become similar to each other; they are now a uniform motion.

Example: we draw a quick circle on paper. This circle is quite unique, because we cannot reproduce it exactly. When we draw another circle, we shall see that it is quite different. It takes a lot of drawing experience and effort to copy the first circle exactly. Now we decide to learn to draw a proper circle because the ones that we have drawn were skewed, not properly round. We draw circles, hundreds of circles, and eventually, we learn to draw a round circle. We can now draw almost the same circle every time, we don't even have to watch it any more.

What we achieve is this: we have learned a general movement, so that we can now perform it routinely, without having to pay much attention to it. We learn habits. We learn to recite some poem, and to play the piano, as a routine.

We also learn, quite involuntarily, to produce abnormal body changes in exactly the same way, if these abnormal patterns persist.

If we are constantly in an alarm response in which our body is geared for possible emergencies that exist only in our fearful fancy, this alarm response will become chronic. The process of chronification means that such a persistent state of abnormal arousal must become fixed in stable bodily pattern; first in persistent functions, later in persistent structural changes. We then see changes appearing such as raised blood pressure, palpitations, and other alterations that indicate the state of fixed (chronic) arousal.

Changes come and go, but if they persist, then they will be laid out into a fixed function, and later in a bodily form. If we wish to rid ourselves of abnormal changes we must practise them away. Undoing bad changes must also be practised.

Practice means regular repetition, and if we are prepared to practise the right changes, they will eventually take the place of the wrong ones. I have stressed the word eventually, because this process of righting, of rectification, takes repetition and time: it is also a process of chronification. Doing it once or twice, or irregularly, is not good enough. We practise the changes systematically and that means regular repetition in a rhythmic pattern.

Examples:

• If a man with high blood pressure sits in meditation for thirty minutes, this will not lower his blood pressure by much. If it does, then it is not usually sustained beyond the duration of the session. If he practises this meditation (it is not true meditation, but merely relaxation) three times daily for at least three weeks, then we may find his blood pressure lowered more persistently. Consistent and systematic practice, a devotion to practice, will be required for this normalising effect to become stable.

This is no different from being given medication. One tablet will not drop the blood pressure, and only after about two weeks of regular tablet taking will the blood pressure be consistently found at a lower level.

• If you walk once across a patch of grass, this should not leave any permanent changes. The trampled grass soon veers back to its previous form. If you walk across the grass in the same direction frequently, you will shape a pathway into the patch.

• When we are stressed, and we learn to relax, the first few sessions will only produce a sense of calm detachment for the duration of the session, and for perhaps an hour or so afterwards. Only by systematic practice can we bring our level of working tension down to normal (below the stress level), for the whole day.

This should also clear up one misconception; you do not have to fear that casual negative thoughts will do you any harm, as so many people seem to think. Only if these bad thoughts are practised systematically, repeated regularly and consistently, can they become harmful.

Sometimes it seems that even with regular practice, nothing is changing. The change comes later, and it may come suddenly. An old story illustrates this well: a man earned his living by breaking big rocks into gravel, which he and his wife then sold. One day he came across a large rock, and tried to crush it. He beat it eighteen times with his heavy hammer, yet the rock would not break. He was ready to give up and look for another, but his wife asked him to give it one last blow, and when he did, the rock fell into pieces. The breaks were already present, but not yet detectable.

Professor J. H. Schultz (who was a professor of neurology and psychiatry at the University of Berlin) began his famous book on autogenic training with the remark that his method of self-relaxation must be regarded as a training: that it requires systematic practice.

This self-generated (auto-genic) method will produce positive changes in us if it is practised with regular repetition. He pointed out that the effect of one hypnotic session is not permanent, that it soon wears off unless it is maintained.

The effect must be kept active by regular supportive practice if we want it to persist. We can see here the principle of biological economy at work: if you want to keep the change, continue to practise it until it is firmly established. Then practise to maintain it.

This is how our body works. A muscle man who stops practising will soon lose his large muscles. If such muscles are not used regularly there is no need for their excessive size, so that they will be efficiently reduced to his regular daily level of activity. This process of downward adjustment in medicine is known as disuse atrophy.

On the other hand, if you regularly lift ever heavier loads, your muscles will increase their size appropriately. This upward adaptation is known as hypertrophy. If we lose one kidney, the regular increase in the workload of the remaining kidney will stimulate it to grow larger, as if to compensate for the loss, and do the work of two.

A musician, athlete, dancer, or other performer, who fails to practise, will soon lose his or her facility, and will require renewed practice to regain it. This is the principle of biological economy that is important to understand. Learned behaviour, routine, and habit, are only practised phenomena: they are formations of change into stable patterns.

It is almost unnecessary to state that everything that happens in the organism is an activity. We must also understand that everything that we see as a structure inside this body is actually an unseen activity. What we perceive as a structure is a slow fixed movement, because this is practical if we have to work on it. We have sense organs for a practical purpose.

Hierarchy of levels of causation. A hierarchy is a kind of pecking order. The emotional mind is the big boss at the top and instructs the body through the nervous system. The organ systems (digestive, circulatory, respiratory, excretory functions) are on a level below the nervous system. Below this layer of organ systems are the organs themselves, and below these organs are the cells that represent the lowest units in the pecking order. Rather than perceiving this as a hierarchy of structures, it is more useful to see it as a pecking order of increasingly smaller functions. Compare this to the pecking order of jobs in the state public service. Instructions for work to be done begin at the top (Premier) and filter down to the ministerial departments, from there to the local councils, and finally to the workers.

The total organism is the original biological unit of change. Any change begins with affecting this entire organism. It is often, and quite wrongly, thought that all changes begin with biochemical changes in the cells, because these cells are supposed to be the biological units of any living system. This is a mistaken notion that has been obtained by an analysis of the living system. Without going into it any deeper here, we may say that: first there was the organism as a whole, and only later came the cell.

An amoeba, for example, is a one-cell organism that performs all the basic functions that, later in evolution, are done by more permanent organs inside the organism. The organism moves, and directs its internal processes appropriately, so that all changes begin in the total organism, and filter downward from the organ systems to the organs, and from these to the cells.

This is important for our understanding that anything that happens, must begin with the emotional mind that guides the organism in its interaction with its environment.

What happens inside the body, with the exception of material accidents, is always determined in this process of interaction with the world. Such interaction is regulated by the emotional mind.

If we want to bring change to the body without overriding the emotional mind by using drugs or surgery, we must always begin with this emotional mind, that is engaged in interaction with its environment. Here is where all our involuntary decisions are made, all those instructions that are aimed at our direct survival.

Here is a schematic picture of the relationship between the emotional mind and the body.

The emotional mind contains the body inside itself, and the nervous system regulates the entire body as the mediator between emotional mind and the rest of the body. The cells are part of the

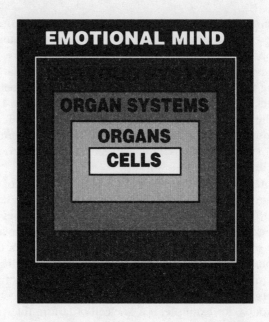

organs, and these, in turn, belong to the organ systems. These organ systems are functions, and we may compare these to government functions such as the post, water and electricity, and transport.

The government decides that there should be a mail service, and this is like an instruction from the emotional mind. The ministry for postal services works out the technical details and this is our nervous system. Special instructions now go to the department for postal services to carry out the function or task of bringing mail around. This can be compared to our circulation system. The function of bringing mail around makes it necessary to have post offices, mail sorting equipment, cars, and so on. The job decides what persons and machinery will be needed to carry it out. These are the organs and cells.

All living systems have two fundamental programs, of which one is the main program, the other a supporting program. The main program is that of interaction, and we are not far wrong when we say that we live to interact, and not the other way around.

The supporting program consists of an inner action-support (interaction-support) program, and an internal life-support program.

We have two fundamental biological needs from which all our other organismic needs have sprouted: the need to interact, and the need to heal. These are profound needs, and if these are not satisfied, the resulting biological frustration must cause considerable harm to the organism.

(a) This is why enduring (chronic) entrapment must always lead to apathy and demoralisation.

(b) This is why the frustration of our need to heal will lead to complications. If the creation of a healing atmosphere is made impossible, so that there is no possibility of recovery in a stress-free zone, we should expect that complications may arise. This need may be frustrated by difficulties that allow no opportunity for resting, by deliberate sabotage, or through anxiety and inhibitions.

An unexpected cause of this frustration is also a too strong reliance on rational logic, because healing, like all other life functions, is governed by emotional logic. If rational logic is sceptical about emotional logic, this may interfere with healing simply because it will not be allowed to start for as long as the rational mind remains actively critical.

We may simplify this as follows: knowledge does not heal, it can only contribute to it. Beliefs (faith is also a belief) heal, because they are based on the same logic as healing. If the belief in your recovery does not come spontaneously, then practise and practise it, until it is established.

Practice is an example of emotional logic. We expect knowledge to be sufficient for instant and enduring change. We expect an insight into a problem to be enough. But it does not work that way, as Freud found out to his initial dismay, because that is only typical of rational logic. Emotional logic says: whatever it is that you wish to change, practise it.

This systematic repetition is essentially a learning process. Sudden healing is rare, and most healing is gradual, and must be supported and maintained by regular practice. This is why hypnotically induced change does not last. To last, it must be kept up for long enough to become permanent.

Healing mode. This is the life-support mode that can only be activated by resting the action-system. We must immobilise our body so that our emotional mind is released from its action-guiding work. As long as this mind is still restless and scattered, however, we cannot expect to be in the healing mode yet. Relieved from its natural task, it is as if it does not know what to do with itself, and casts about for something, anything, to do. Well, we give it something to do: we give it one single thing to keep itself occupied with, and this should settle it more.

Our emotional mind is a restless mind by nature, a mind that is ordinarily preoccupied with leading the organism in action, and it is an impatient mind for that reason. If it has nothing to do, and it is not time for sleeping, it becomes fretful and behaves like a bored child that starts to think up all kinds of mischief. We must give it something to do to settle it more if we wish to relax.

We can settle this emotional mind in two ways:

• By keeping it busy with relaxing the body. As our muscles become limp when we relax our action system, the rest of the body quietens down, and the emotional mind gradually subsides. With the body relaxed, the mind is at ease.

• By keeping it busy with one single monotonous activity.

This may be mental activity, such as silently repeating a single word, a phrase, a short prayer; counting the breathing, or accompanying it with the thought 'in and out and in and out . . .'

This may also be achieved by a rhythmic monotonous movement of the body, rhythmically weaving or rocking back and forth while sitting or standing, by walking or by running. We must make sure that this is a rhythmic and monotonous activity.

(i) the movement must always be the same movement, lest the mind becomes interested and aroused by the changing activity.

(ii) it must have a rhythm that will occupy the attentive mind, so it holds the mind spellbound, as it were.

The two can be combined, so that we rhythmise the movement.

Examples:

Watch the breathing movements of your abdomen and accompany this breathing action by thinking: in – out – in – out.

Alternatively: in-and-out-and-in-and-out . . . and so on.

Other methods, counting the breathing:

• one count per breath: in-one—out-two . . . etc;

• several counts per breath: in-two-three — out-two-three.

Weave back and forth while sitting limp in a chair, leaning over a little for stability, and rhythmise the movements with breathing and counting:

- on breathing out, weave and count: out-two-three-four.
- on breathing in, weave and count: in-two-three-four.

Concentrate your attentive mind on the feeling in the tip of the tongue. Purse your lips around it if you need to make that feeling stronger, so you can concentrate on it more easily. You have thus brought your mind to the feeling, and now keep it there. Hold it there by thinking one thought only such as: 'tip-of-tongue, tip-of-tongue' in rapid succession, so that the mind has no chance of escaping. This will settle it, so that it will gradually stay with the feeling, and not let it go to think something else, something more interesting.

Treat your emotional mind like you would train a waiting child to sit still and behave, by giving it something to do.

In short, to settle the emotional mind, keep it busy with one single thing, a thought or some movement that is repeated in a regular and monotonous rhythm. This is a hypnotic rhythm, and we use it in self-relaxation as a form of self-hypnosis.

Our emotional mind is an attentive mind. It must focus on the job at hand, and by such focusing it cuts out everything else that has nothing useful to do with this present job. In a room full of people we can keep up a conversation with someone only by blocking out all other voices.

When we finish some activity, and we are idle for the moment, our emotional mind slackens its attention. All sorts of unconnected thoughts, feelings, images, and memories, will drift into our consciousness. Because our emotional mind is now slack and unfocused, our consciousness will be dim, and we feel somewhat drowsy.

This is also what happens as soon as we manage to unhitch our attentive mind from its action-guiding task, as we begin to relax. We must now focus this attentive (emotional) mind by concentrating it on one single thought or feeling, while the body remains relaxed and motionless.

What are the factors that are needed for healing?

(i) The *vis medicatrix naturae*, that spontaneous healing power of nature, on which all healing is based.

(ii) Assisting this natural healing power.

(a) Through medical and/or surgical therapy.

(b) Through personal commitment to supporting this natural healing power to do its work by not standing in its way, and by actively assisting it. This positive self-support is an essential factor in healing.

We shall now concentrate on the last factor: the contribution that we ourselves can make towards our assisted healing. What we need for this active personal contribution is the following:

(a) Rest for recuperation in a stress-free zone.

(b) Relaxation and visualisation to optimise recuperation.

(c) Taking active charge of the situation.

Chapter Twenty-one

RELAXATION

Animals can think, but are limited to practical thinking. They have a practical intelligence; their emotional mind is strictly geared to action. A chimpanzee, for example, can use a stick to reach a banana which is beyond its outstretched arms. This practical intelligence is entirely in the service of survival.

If the animal is not concretely involved with action, then no practical thinking will be needed. When its body is motionless at rest, practical thinking stops as the animal become drowsy and, perhaps, begins to dream impractical dreams.

Only human beings, who have the extra ability for abstraction, can think 'unnecessarily', as far as survival is concerned. We have the ability to think theoretically: to think and imagine beyond practical needs. This is an ability to look beyond the practical here and now, and it can be a luxury or a burden, depending on the content of these thoughts.

On the positive side theoretical thinking is responsible for all progress. But it also has a negative aspect to it: it can imagine harm that goes beyond anything that a merely practical animal is capable of inventing.

We may continue thinking even if there is no practical need for it. We are sitting quietly, having a rest, and may be enjoying it, but we are still fuming about an argument that happened yesterday. Our rest-for-recuperation period is now almost wasted. We can even think of one thing, while we are doing something else. Animals fully concentrate on what they are doing. Only the human organism can fight intergalactic wars while having a shower.

The upshot of this splitting of our attention is, of course, a reduced efficiency. Half our mind is concentrated on doing one thing here and now while the other half is busy elsewhere. It is either occupied with something totally irrelevant, or it is worrying about failing at what we are doing, and hampering our efficiency in the process. We can be half-hearted about a decision, and we can also be half-minded about its execution, so that we are not fully concentrated on it. Its efficiency must therefore suffer. If we want to visualise effectively, we must concentrate fully on the task; we must be full-minded about it.

We can stop action in order to think theoretically in a useful and positive way. We stop (action) to think, and this ability to turn away from the here and now of doing allows us to plan ahead or analyse the past. This is done either for the sake of knowledge alone, or to find some practical use for it.

Our capacity for abstract thinking makes it possible for us to turn away from the practical world of the here and now, and to enter a world of theoretical imagination or emotional fantasy.

This same ability makes it possible to think rationally, but also allows us to indulge in impractical (unrealistic) emotional fantasies. Only the human being can deliberately carry over from the past into the present: we can carry grudges and brood over past wrongs and imagined problems that have no practical value. Only a human being can become a TCP. Animals are limited to being practical.

Human beings have been blessed with a powerfully creative imagination, but we have been unable to make more positive use of it. Because we have never been properly educated in its use, we handle the creative tool awkwardly, and we may use it wrongly, so that it becomes a harmful burden instead. We let our emotional imagination run riot because we have not learned to control it. Our emotional mind is in overdrive and we feel helpless against it, and fear what it might create for us.

If a dog is resting, its practical thinking function is silent because there is no action going on. When an adult human being is resting, its body may be at rest but the emotional mind is still active and usually running unchecked. The emotional mind of the human being is more advanced and versatile than that of animals but in that greater flexibility lies also the danger of becoming uncontrolled and over-active. Most of us find it difficult, if not impossible, to slow down our thinking mind, let alone stop it.

We have learned to think and imagine, but not how to stop

these activities, so the quality of our recuperation is endangered. Recuperation requires our emotional mind to be passive and neutral, so that it is no longer interested in the outer world of action. This mind must let go of its practical preoccupation with being active, its readiness for getting involved in action. This active attitude must change into a passive attitude. This requires a mental stand that is totally uninterested in any kind of action, in doing or imagining it, so that the organism may recuperate.

Our emotional mind can be made passive in two ways; we can do it either by becoming inactive and motionless, or by finding some emotionally neutral and monotonous activity to occupy it. This mental or bodily activity must be regular and monotonous, unchanging, because any change stimulates us, and arouses our active interest.

We do not have to stop thinking for the purpose of recovery. We only need to bundle our attention and to concentrate it on one single neutral thought, body sensation, or activity. We should therefore learn to make our emotional mind single-minded, so we have merely one single thing (thought, body feeling, or action) in our mind. This mind may come to rest in that way, by keeping it occupied with a single neutral and unvarying activity.

As long as the emotional mind finds something interesting to focus on, it remains in an active attitude or mode. While this mind is in this active mode, our internal servicing system cannot start. It must wait until the mind moves into its passive mode. Our self-servicing system cannot begin its work while uncontrolled thinking is going on because irrelevant thoughts and worries can only interfere with its functions.

If our mind is not resting by being still, or by concentration on one single neutral thought, it is prone to invasion by all kinds of irrelevant and unconnected thoughts, memories, and feelings. Our attention is now in a distracted state and open to stray thoughts, memories, and other elements from our inner world. Conflicting emotional directions may now be passed down to the body, instructions that may have nothing to do with internal servicing.

Before we relax, we must make up our mind. What is it that we want: regulation of action or defence and healing? It must be either one or the other. We can't have both. Effective action and healing are mutually exclusive activities in the same way that you can't drive your car and expect your mechanics to service it at the same time. The two activities don't mix. Internal servicing must wait patiently until we decide to rest, to adopt a passive attitude. Practical action requires an active mode, while relaxation (and healing) takes place in a passive mode.

In relaxation and also during action an unfocused emotional mind can be a problem: imagine walking out on an angry confrontation, and then brooding over it while you walk. One set of instructions – for walking – goes to your muscle system. Another set of instructions which are related to fighting over the argument, and that have nothing to do with walking, also arrives at your muscles. The muscle system is now confused about these two conflicting sets of instructions, and tries to incorporate both in the same activity. We should not be surprised, therefore, when we feel exhausted and aching after the walk-in-anger. One set works like a brake on the other, so that our movements are very inefficient.

RELAXING THE BODY TO USE THE MIND

If we wish to visualise more effectively, we must first learn to concentrate the emotional mind on a job that is not action. For this, we need to relax the body first. Why must we relax the body first? Keep in mind that our organism has been designed and built for action, and that both our emotional mind and body are geared to practical doing. If we now want to use the emotional mind for other purposes, such as using it in free fantasy, we must do two things:

We must first release the body from its natural gearing to action, from its action-guiding task. As long as this body remains tense, it stays interested in the outside world, and fit and eager to interact with it. Every sight and every sound, every touch and feel of this world will excite the organism, and invite it to spring to action. This describes our emotional mind in its active attitude: ready to guide the body in instant survival behaviour. The stimulation of our sense organs arouses us, and mobilises our organism for immediate action.

How do we manage to direct our attention away from the outside world? By closing our eyes to this world of sights, and by lying or sitting motionless, so we cannot feel the world of textures.

In this way we prevent sensory contact with it as much as we can. We can't see the world, we can't feel it, and only our ears are still open to it. This allows our emotional mind to lose interest, and to shift into its passive mode. We learn to ignore incoming sounds later, as we relax our body more, and concentrate better.

We help this process of turning away from the outside world by finding a quiet room. We darken it and close its doors. Now we find the most comfortable position for our body, so that we shall not be distracted by unnecessary stimulation. We adopt a symmetrical position in bed (or in a chair), lying (sitting) with the elbows and knees slightly bent, so that there is no tension in them. We support the arms on the bed or chair if possible, or we may rest them on our lap.

We now immobilise this body completely. We release it from its action-orientation. It doesn't have to do anything for a while; it is now inactive, off-duty.

We can experience the usual action-gearing of the body quite clearly as we relax. We feel vaguely uneasy, even guilty, as if we should be doing something useful. We have a feeling that we are wasting precious time, as if we should be more active. We can now almost hear the silent voices of Mother Nature and those of our parents saying: 'Get up, get up, don't just waste valuable time by doing nothing, get up and be productive.'

Sitting still and doing nothing goes against our primitive natural grain, which is that of being and staying active, and only resting in order to go back to work. However, this is a primitive urge. In sitting still we may exercise our highest, our most sophisticated, human capacity. As we sit relaxed, our emotional mind matures further; it learns to become patient. It is much harder to sit still than to be active, in the same way that being mature is more demanding than being childish.

We all had to learn to become patient as we grew up, and we only need to look at children to realise – and remember – how difficult a task that is. Animals and children are by nature impatient, they are urgent creatures, itching to be in action.

There is nothing more difficult than to sit still, to wait, to exercise patience, and to refrain from jumping into action. Maturity is the ability to be patient, and being patient implies tolerance and endurance.

Our answer to this sense of guilt on sitting still should be: we are not wasting time by relaxing, we are investing in the quality of our future . . . by recovering better, and by becoming more mature.

The initial uncomfortable feeling of guilt will fade after a while. As with any other feeling, it passes more quickly when we relax.

Feelings are like waves; they come and go. Feelings have been organised, designed, to come on like a wave of urgency, and then to pass, because that is practical for the guidance of an organism that has to cope with constantly changing situations. Our feelings come and go, because our situations come and go.

Normal feelings may come but they must also go. By tensing, we make them stronger, because this is practical for our survival action. We are much more tense and sensitive, and our emotions are much stronger, more urgent, when we cross a busy road than when we sit in the garden reading a book.

When we don't need feelings or don't even want them, we relax to reduce their strength. A practical rule of thumb is: tense up and you double pain, relax and you halve it. What goes for pain, also goes for any other feeling, such as itching, anger, and anxiety.

Feelings that persist are usually abnormal feelings. Feelings that don't pass tell us that the situation is not changing as it should, that it is being prevented from developing naturally. Pain, anxiety, anger, depression, and so on are feelings that usually come to warn that some problem situation exists, so that we may deal with it. If these pass, all is well. When they persist, however, there is something wrong. We have here a continuing problem that needs to be resolved. This kind of situation, as we have seen, may be a trap.

When the body is totally relaxed, we have no need for feelings and sensitivity, because we are not doing anything right now.

As we relax our body, we release it from any need to be active and practical. We release our organism from its need to be tense, and from the need to have emotions and to be sensitive. By relaxing this body, we also uncouple our emotional mind from the need to guide this body in practical action, so that we can turn our mind to the task of creative visualisation. We need a passive mind for this task: a passive emotional mind is a pacified mind.

We can easily check this because, as we rest, images come up that have little or nothing to do with the guiding of action. We experience such irrelevant and disconnected images both in relaxation and in dreaming. The only real difference between the dream reality and our waking reality is this; in the dream we have been released from the need to be practical. Our mind is now no longer reduced and bound to being only practical, so that it is relatively free in its fancy. In the dream we are no longer limited to being realistic in a practical world.

We can now fly like a bird, be the ruler of the universe, we can be anything and do anything. It is as if we have left our practical body behind, so that our highly creative emotional mind begins its tale of free fantasy. It is uncommon to retain the practical action-form of the body in the dream. If we do, then this is usually just before waking, when our organism is tensing up and preparing itself for the practical working day. At this time, our dreams are usually more real, more life-like.

We need this freedom from practical needs for visualisation. It allows us to break through any abnormal inhibitions that we might have about the topic we wish to visualise. Inhibiting attitudes become activated by a tension response. At rest they lie dormant in the mind. Visualisation in relaxation mobilises these attitudes, but our relaxed state prevents them from overwhelming us. We can now correct them. This is why visualisation is a useful technique in treating inhibited personalities who suffer from emotional restraints.

Such inhibitions have their origin in the childhood emotional imagination, and we have seen that in that period the child is still unable to tell the adult difference between reality and imagination. For the child, there is no such difference. When we talk about unrealistic fears, therefore, we indicate those of the adult, and not of the child whose fears are real enough in their childhood setting. Only if these persist into adulthood, do they become unrealistic, because they have not been changed.

Mr TCP will thus be able to relieve himself from his voodoo, which is a dangerous restraint on his survival, by relaxing his emotional mind that is narrowed, and focused on dying.

How do we relax our body? First and foremost by letting our muscles go completely limp. We should learn to do this systematically, to follow a practical pattern, such as we shall describe in the following pages.

We have so many muscles that it would be impossible to relax every individual muscle. Our body is geared to action, and we have an action system, and a support system to look after it. We only need to relax this action system.

- one face for communicating with the world;
- two arms for operating on the world;
- two legs for moving around in the world.

That's all we need to relax. We simply allow these parts to go limp for a while, and then encourage them to become even more limp by using our imagination: vividly imagine your arms and legs being completely limp and floppy.

The rest of the body, everything housed in the trunk (between the shoulders and hips), consists of the support system for our action system. This supporting system will merely follow the instructions that reach it from the action system at the front line with the outer world, so that it must relax automatically, as we immobilise our action system.

THE SIGNS OF SUCCESSFUL RELAXATION

The experience of our relaxed body is entirely different from that of our body in action. We are familiar with our body in action, because we have experienced this since our childhood. The relaxed body presents us with an entirely different way of experiencing ourselves, and the various signs and symptoms of successful relaxation add up to this different experience of our relaxed body. This body is in calm repose while we are awake rather than asleep:

(a) A comfortable feeling of heaviness in the limbs: our limbs become heavy, because limp muscles are heavy and feel heavy. When a child wants to be picked up, he will strain towards you, and this makes him light. If he is unwilling, he instantly goes limp in your arms, and you then find out how heavy this uncooperative child is. Children are also heavy when asleep.

When we wake up in the morning, we spontaneously activate our body, we make it fit-for-action by tensing up. We stretch and yawn and otherwise mobilise our working body. As we stretch, we activate our antigravity muscles; those are muscles that keep us upright and feeling light-and-fit for action. Imagine standing tall and raising your arms to the sky, and stretching towards it, as if you are about to fly up. This will tense the antigravity muscles, so that you can clearly feel them.

By allowing them to become limp, we lose that lightness. It is replaced by a sense of heaviness. We also lose that sense of fitness, we feel at ease instead.

The face has thin muscles. They haven't enough volume to feel heavy. Instead, the face feels like a smooth, bland and impersonal mask. This is the experience of a face at rest and at ease: a face that is not in use. When the jaw muscles are relaxed, there will be space between the teeth, so that the relaxed face feels longer.

(b) A comfortable feeling of laziness: this is the feeling of ease; it is the reluctance to get going that we experience when we wake up from a deep and good quality sleep. We feel relaxed, comfortable, cosy and quite loath to stir, because our muscles have switched off.

To get our organism going again, we must call our muscles back to work. We stretch and yawn until we feel fit; light and clear-headed for action.

(c) A feeling of fuzziness: when the body relaxes, it no longer needs to be sensitive, so it becomes half-way numb, which is one of the reasons for halving the strength of any feeling.

When the body does not have to be active, when it is resting, it no longer needs to have a body sense (body-image) that is geared to action. We don't have to keep track of where our arms, face, or any other part of the body, are located, while we are at rest.

Our normal body image is a practical one. When we are fit and active, we are clearly aware of the shape and position of our active parts. We need that awareness for practical work. Our organism, as we said, works on the principle of biological economy. You save energy by switching off a light you don't need. For the same reason, your body switches off its active guiding image when you are not moving about. It saves energy. Working tension is needed to keep up this action-oriented body image.

The loss of this practical body experience is useful to test your progress in relaxation. You feel it as a shapeless, warm, tingling fuzziness in which you have lost track of the various parts. The loss of the normal action-shape of our body tells us that the body has now been disconnected from its need for action. This partially numb sensation is one of the reasons why pain, and other forms of discomfort, are lessened by relaxing.

When you have finished relaxing, reactivate the body to bring back this action image by taking a deep breath and stretching.

This calls your rested muscles back to work.

Pain is not merely a sensation that warns of danger, it is at the same time an emotion that is associated with fear of harm. When we relax, our emotions fade as our sensitivity decreases and pain is reduced both as a sensation and an emotion. Pain, anxiety, and tension, belong together in one group, and so do comfort, calm and relaxation (muscle limpness).

As long as we remain active, we need to be orientated in the world around us, and in the location of our own action body in it. When we now are motionless, we have no further need to be orientated in the outer world. We give this up as soon as we close our eyes and lie still. Now, by rights, we should feel slightly disorientated. We may experience a sense of floating, turning, tilting, and other such disorientation sensations, as we abandon our practical orientation towards the world and towards our own body.

(d) A cosy sense of warmth: later still, as we manage to relax further, we have a sense of warmth that envelops us. Our skin warms up. This happens when the blood in our skin is no longer diverted to the muscles for the sake of action. It flows back into the blood vessels under the skin, and this is much like switching on an electric blanket to warm the bed covers.

When we are truly relaxed, we should experience this welcome warmth. It will merge with the feeling of fuzziness to become a fuzzy warmth: a comforting warmth that can soothe painful areas of the body. We feel protected by this warmth, as if cocooned in a shelter.

(e) Settling of our breathing and pulse: as our action system becomes immobilised, our respiratory and circulation systems must reduce their level of activity so that our breathing and pulse rates begin to slow down.

Our digestive system that shuts down during action, now comes alive again. Digestive juices begin to flow. We notice this as a flow of saliva in the mouth as we relax. Just swallow it as it comes. Our stomach and bowels resume their contractions. We may hear this as a happy rumble in the abdomen as we relax.

(f) A sense of ease: when our body is limp and motionless, we experience a sense of ease. This is what we usually mean by a sense of calm, detachment, equanimity, tranquillity, serenity, bliss or peacefulness. It is fundamentally a profound feeling of ease that now replaces the feeling of fitness of an active body. In a relaxed state we do not feel fit in well-being, but at ease in well-being. The body is now no longer an instrument for action, but merely a fuzzy cloud of feeling.

There are now no practical or theoretical distinctions between body and mind. They merge with each other into one experience of ease. This condition is called immersion or absorption, and it is the starting point for the search for liberation (mystic union). This search requires profound meditation, and it does not concern us here because it is not necessary for recovery. It is postgraduate stuff.

These six points are six aspects of one and the same relaxation experience. They are all described in Schultz's method of autogenic training, although not in this particular sequence. Autogenic training is, without any doubt, the most efficient method for self-relaxation that is available.

Chapter Twenty-two

THE EXPERIENCE OF RELAXATION

As we relax our body and free the emotional mind from its task of guiding the body in action, we also automatically switch on our internal servicing (healing) system.

The emotional mind, now relieved of its natural guiding task, gradually loses its impatient, action-urging character, and becomes calm and detached: at ease. The body is now no longer bound to practical action, and can no longer produce feelings of tension-for-action. Instead, as we saw, it creates in us a sense of ease in well-being.

We now feel warm, secure, and sheltered. All our action-geared emotions and sensation have faded away, so that we experience a sense of easy neutrality: the world of action seems remote, distant, less important. If we go deeper from here, we shall feel that nothing seems to matter any more, that nothing is important. If anything still seems to matter, it means we are still hooked into the action-world. We have not relaxed deeply enough, and our emotional mind is therefore still geared to action.

In relaxation, we are in a tension-free zone, and therefore also in a stress-free zone. This is the proper atmosphere for internal servicing of the major kind: for maximum repair and maintenance. By staying in this condition for a while, we allow healing to take place that is of far better quality than the minor service that we usually get in our ordinary uneasy sleep and rest.

We shall find that thinking does not stop very easily. Even when the body is already quite limp and relaxed, the mind is still active, thinking of this and that. Uninvited thoughts keep popping into our mind to seduce us into following them up. This is an active emotional mind that involuntarily brings up such thoughts, images and feelings.

We find that we have very little control over this coming and going of the thoughts, images, or feelings, that are no longer action-bound and practical. There is no need to stop thinking. We only need to guide this activity into the right direction, and that is: relaxation followed by visualisation. We channel our thinking in a useful direction.

As we relax, our thinking process will change its character. Active thinking in terms of words (concepts) now makes place for passive imagery: picture thinking. This also happens when we have idle day dreams, and when we dream at night. Were we to relax deeper still, then even these images would disappear; they would be replaced by feelings. (Even these feelings will eventually fade away, but that need not concern us here.) We only need to relax enough to unhook our thinking from its practical preoccupation, and then use it for visualising.

Relaxing in this manner is a self-initiated and self-directed process, and the rational mind keeps an eye on our progress, sitting in the passenger's seat, and doing the navigation and self-correction. When an interesting thought pops into our mind, our emotional mind is inclined to pursue it, but our watchful rational mind says: Hey, stop that, come back to relaxing and stay here.

As we begin, our impatient emotional mind tends to wander off, and we patiently guide it back to the job at hand. We need it for relaxing and visualising. This happens particularly if we are tense, stressed, or tired. These states make relaxation more difficult, and it is often useful to rest a while before beginning the relaxation process.

We adopt a strategy to prevent the wandering mind from going off in all directions. We focus this mind on one single thought so that, instead of thinking many different thoughts one after another, we now limit it to one single thought that we repeat rapidly, over and over again, until the mind settles on the job, and is less inclined to wander off. Don't try to stop these thoughts, because the effort will only tense you up.

It is usually quite easy to bring the mind to the area that we wish to concentrate on, but it is much more difficult to make it stay there. The rapid repetition of the single thought will keep the mind focused on the job until it settles (notice here the stabilising effect of repetition).

Imagine, if you will, that every single thought is a stitch with which we apply the mind to the area; a close stitch will make it stay bound until it begins to calm down. We can then slow down, and even cease the thought altogether.

Focus your attention on the tip of your tongue, as described in chapter twenty. If necessary, tighten your lips over it a little, or push it against the back of the teeth, to make the feeling stronger and easier to hold onto.

Now concentrate your mind on the feeling in the tip. Bring it there, and keep it there, as described, until the mind settles more reliably on this feeling. Now your mind is single-mindedly concentrated on the feeling by the use of a constant single thought. This is excellent relaxation practice, because it relaxes you in the process, so that you should feel quite at ease when you have finished with it.

Self-relaxation is not difficult to learn, but it is best when it is taught by a competent practitioner. Once it is learned, it has to be practised. It must be rehearsed with consistent and painstaking devotion: with the same diligence with which you would practise to learn to play an instrument, or learn to perform an athletic feat.

Relaxation is a performance, visualising is a performance, and your recovery is just as much a performance. Rehearse properly for a perfect performance.

You don't have to relax deeply to increase the efficiency of internal servicing; nature never demands that. Going deeper in order to still the emotional mind completely is useful only if you wish to search for mystic union. If so, then you must seek isolation from the social world. There is no need to still the emotional mind for the purposes of effective visualisation. All we need to do is to unhook it from action, and to channel it in the right direction.

Relaxation reduces the strength (intensity) of all feelings and sensations, so that we feel calm (emotionally neutral) and fuzzy (reduced sensitivity: we are halfway numb). In this way we can now overcome inhibitions that were too strong before. Inhibitions are also feelings; they are played out in freezing attitudes or other blocking activities.

We may now work on such negative feelings; we remove them in a visualised situation and rehearse this until it works in the actual one. We change negative images into positive ones, and this is no different from the practice of mental rehearsal of professional performers. An example may make this clear.

A phobia is a strong and abnormal anxiety about something. To confront this phobia without further ado, as is sometimes advised, is not a good idea, because you are likely to fail. If you want to learn wrestling you don't begin by challenging the giant mauler. You had better practise on a little brother or sister, or you may lose confidence and give up.

Relaxation reduces the strength of the phobia. Once this phobic intensity has been brought down to a more manageable size you can learn to overcome it by visualising a successful struggle. Raw confrontation is likely to makes you lose the fight. It is much better to rehearse it mentally first, to practise it in visualisation during relaxation.

If we have a phobia about the cancer monster and we apply the same method, then this monster shrinks to the size of a creature that we feel fit to fight.

Relaxation is not merely something to make you feel better: it activates an intense healing process, provided it is performed correctly. Nor is relaxation limited to coping with cancer. It is equally effective in any other kind of illness, and in the management of stress, and any kind of discomfort, such as pain. It is also efficient in reducing pre- and post-operative stress, for example, so that it improves the quality and speed of recovery. It supports mother nature's medicine, and even enhances it. Relaxation prepares us for coping better with life and most of its problems, by reducing the strength of normal and abnormal emotions and sensitivity to a more manageable size.

What relaxation provides us with is, in short, what Reinhold Niebuhr prayed for (quoted in an earlier chapter): the strength to change that which can be changed, the courage to accept that which cannot be changed, and the wisdom to tell one from the other.

RELAXATION IN PRACTICE

Complete muscle relaxation produces a state of immobility that changes the quality of the mind as well as of the body. It deactivates the body and therefore automatically activates internal servicing.

It also clears the mind of its natural-primitive preoccupation with action. If we wish to cross a busy road, for example, we must tense up to a good level of working tension. This primes us, both bodily and mentally, for effective action. Should we want to use our mind for more sophisticated work, however, we clear it first by relaxing. We tense up to go hunting, but we relax to clear our mind for free thinking.

The degree of immobility that we must produce to effect change can only be achieved by training, by methodical and diligent practice. When the body is freed from its action-gearing, the emotional mind is free to change. Feelings lose their strength and urgency, so that they can no longer have a strong hold over us. We let them fade away. This is the proper way to deal with anger, for example. Don't bottle it up, because you will suffer. Don't lash out hysterically at your social environment either, because it will make others suffer, and you may feel guilty and ashamed. Relax and learn to let it fade away. You can't be angry when you are relaxed. You can't be calm and have strong feelings at the same time.

Negative feelings can change, and by regular and persistent practice, the body can also be made to change its negative habits because such habits are merely stiffened feelings that have been stabilised by practice. They can change, but only by systematic practice.

To practise systematically, we must have some kind of order in the method. Recall that our organism is designed for action, and that it has a leading head, two arms and two legs for this purpose. What we have to do, is relieve it from its natural task, so that we follow this method:

First, we de-activate the leading head. This means that we must de-activate the sensory organs. We darken the room and close our eyes, we close the doors to shut out most sound, and we lie still and comfortable to prevent ourselves from becoming excited by feeling around. Now we de-activate the face, which is the organ for communicating with the world. We don't need to use it for a while. Take some time to relax your face: the face is the most overworked part of the body because it is in constant use. We use it when we speak and think (thinking is silent speech and thoughts are silent voices), and when we express emotions. The more tense we are, the more we increase the activity of the face until it becomes like a tight fist. We don't even feel it any more because we have become so used to walking around with a clenched fist for a face, that we take this for granted. Having allowed this leading head to rest, we must now turn to our limbs:

Second, we de-activate our arms and legs. We can do this by letting them go limp and loose. Like our face, they are tools for action that we don't need for a while, so that we can abandon them. Successful de-activation is signalled by the feeling of a lazy heaviness in the limbs, a mask-like feeling in the face, and a general sense of fuzziness in the entire body, with a sense of calm detachment and ease in the emotional mind.

Because we let go of our world of practical action, we must also abandon our orientation in it, which is now unnecessary anyway. Don't be surprised, therefore, to experience a certain degree of disorientation while you close your eyes and lie still to relax. It usually begins when we close our eyes, but we have become so used to this that we don't pay it any attention.

As we begin to relax, we may feel the disoriented feelings of a relaxing body. Our muscles become limp as we turn away from the outside world and as we abandon all ideas of action. We may experience feelings of floating, turning, levitating, tilting, and sinking, as the body loses its action shape. This happens normally every night when we go to sleep, but we have no awareness of it, because we are already too drowsy.

Don't be afraid of these feelings, because they are merely the normal feelings of a relaxing body. Enjoy the experience while you can because these sensations usually disappear with more practice.

Sometimes suppressed emotions which are contained emotions that we cannot bring ourselves to express, burst out into the open as we relax our suppressing attitude. They come out with talking, crying, laughing, twitching, shivering and so on. Let them out freely, because they are better out than in, and the relaxed state is a safe place for their free expression.

Chapter Twenty-three

HEALING BEYOND TREATMENT: USING VISUALISATION

What is the difference between treatment and healing? Treatment is what you receive from someone else and healing is what you do yourself. A wound, for example, is treated by your doctor who merely cleanses it and stitches its edges together. Such doctoring only promotes healing.

A typical confusion between healing and treatment often takes place when a course of chemotherapy or radiotherapy has finished. The patient may ask: 'What happens to me next? Now that this treatment is finished, who is going to treat me?' The answer is: 'The treatment may be over, but you go on with your task of healing.'

A therapist treats but the body heals. The mind supports this healing routine by taking active charge of it.

(a) Remove any physical and emotional obstacles to healing. Boost your general health and get rid of any helplessness and powerlessness.

(b) Shift into the healing mode (relaxation).

(c) Enhance healing through visualisation.

The next five chapters describe how that can be achieved.

The emotional mind can be turned to healing as soon as we have released it from its practical connection with direct action. Action-gearing narrows our mind to a practical mind, it makes the mind fit only for practical interaction with the world, so that we must first learn to free it from its natural obsession with action. We must rest this mind from action, if we wish to use it for rational thinking or free emotional fantasy, or for visualisation in service of recovery. We must first create an action-free and stress-free zone for healing.

In the state of relaxation, we extend our voluntary influence over the body. This deliberate influence is normally limited to what we need for direct and practical interaction with the outer world. We can decide to run across the road, eat a pear or hold our breath for a short while, for example, but we cannot reduce, or speed up, our pulse rate, ease pain, or become warm, at will, by voluntary decision because all this is not necessary for practical survival.

Yet we do have the potential to influence many functions that are not ordinarily accessible because they are not part of our practical everyday needs. This potential is like a reserve of influence that we can call on, if we are not in our normal action-geared (practical, waking) adult mode of consciousness.

In our ordinary everyday activities we only exercise those muscles that we need for such activities. For example, manual labour requires other muscle combinations than wordprocessing, and the level of need determines how large and strong the used muscles have to be. Our unused muscles shrink to their resting size and form a muscle reserve that we ordinarily do not need to call on.

A secretary will have problems with manual labour and a road worker will find typing quite awkward. The other kind of work, the non-ordinary kind for the job, will have to be learned by systematic practice.

To develop the appropriate bodily or mental muscle, we must go through a learning process. Proper hypnotic treatment is, in fact, just such mental muscle building. Autogenic training was created by Professor Schultz for this purpose. It is a very effective method of self-hypnosis that, once learned, can be practised without further supervision. The improvement may be kept up by the subject herself. The key to such self-improvement is passive concentration, and we shall take this up later. It is with this passively focused concentration that we open up our reserve capacity.

Gaining access to this reserve is not done by using so-called will power. This has no power, it is merely a decision by the rational mind that is sitting in the passenger's seat. It is fairly useless, because the rational mind does not sit at the controls. Our New Year resolutions are witness to that. They last only as long as we remember them; a day or a week.

The rational mind can make a plan, but must submit that plan to the emotional mind for its execution. It can only advise. Getting the emotional mind to cooperate is the trick. We can do this by means of relaxation and appropriate visualisation training.

APPROPRIATE VISUALISATION: CREATING APPROPRIATE SITUATIONS

Visualisation is the art of creating appropriate situations.

How do we reduce our pulse rate, without using drugs? Willing it to slow down is useless, and it may even bring about the reverse. We achieve it by relaxing our mind and body. This drops the rate automatically from seventy-eight beats per minute to about sixty. The condition of relaxed immobility (we can also be tense and motionless) creates an appropriate situation for a slow pulse rate. If we are not moving, we need only little oxygen and fuel, so that circulation and breathing functions slow down to a minimum level of activity. This is our resting level. Our pulse and breathing rates dwindle to an appropriate level.

How can we speed up our pulse rate? Normally, this happens when we are excited by an actual danger or a sexual situation, or any other situation that arouses us. It is not always necessary to be in an actual (real) situation. A visualised (imagined) situation will do. The thought or picture that we have, if we can make it sufficiently vivid and dreamlike, will produce the desired effect, such as a raised pulse rate. Any situation of arousal is appropriate for it.

Fooling the body. Why is it that a visualised situation can be so effective in achieving results? The child's emotional mind cannot yet make clear distinctions between what is a practical reality and what is imagination, so her body will respond in the much same way to what she sees and what she imagines in fantasy. This goes on until the child's emotional mind has been sufficiently trained in making practical distinctions between reality and imagination. Her capacity for imagination becomes increasingly idle as the child grows up, and lies mostly unused with the average adult. Later the child also learns to make theoretical distinctions, but we need not concern ourselves with that here.

Our adult emotional mind has been trained in being practical when we are awake, as we saw in the previous chapters. It has learned to ignore our imagination if it is not of practical survival value. That is why it is necessary that we relax. We must first release our emotional mind from this practical task of selective judging if we want to make use of it for other purposes, those that do not demand immediate action.

In stress, this mind also loses its practical guiding quality, so that here also, our creative imagination becomes effective in producing bodily changes. Unfortunately, these are negative images and bodily changes, harmful creations that have been motivated by enduring helplessness, anxiety, and anger.

A European yogi (as he called himself) once confided that he raised his pulse rate, not by willpower, as he first claimed, but by visualising himself in a danger situation in which a raised pulse rate would be appropriate. He vividly imagined an appropriate situation of losing a fight with a stronger enemy who was pushing him over the edge of a cliff.

We use the same method; we visualise an appropriate situation; this is a setting in which the effect we are after would occur naturally. Any image that arouses us will speed up our pulse, in the same way as the visualisation of a warming situation will make us feel warm. Any image that settles us, such as a calm, restful, and quiet beach or garden will reduce our pulse and breathing rates.

The situation must be an emotionally charged one, if it is to arouse us. A neutral situation has the effect of settling us, because it lacks any promise or threat of immediate action. Depending on the effect that we are after, we should create a situation with a certain tone: pleasant if we wish to relax further, or exciting if we want to be aroused.

This tone (atmosphere) is a general situational tone in which all images are embedded, so that they are in harmony with it. If you write about a pleasant garden, the atmosphere of pleasantness that you have thus set, will now determine the quality of the images that will appear in it. These will be in harmony with the feeling tone of pleasantness unless you wish to shock by creating a contrast. One effective way of creating colour harmony, is to brush a colour on to a canvas, and then paint other colours into this wet colour, so they all take up a little of the main colour or mother-colour. This harmonises them.

Compare this to dream situations: if we wish to understand the dream our first question should be: what is its setting, and the main feeling-tone that is present? The images that appear in it will have the same feeling of the setting, and are merely an elaboration of it.

The bleak setting of a narrow, dark, and desolate street in a dream is a direct expression of our state of mind. It mirrors our captive and anxious mind in this visualised state. Of the almost unlimited possibilities for richness and pleasantness that are available to us in free dreaming, we were limited to creating such a dismal setting.

We could have been rulers of the universe, yet our unfree mind could only dream up an existence in a narrow and dark street, because it was so bound by anxiety and insecurity.

What happens involuntarily in a natural situation, we can also make happen in a visualised situation, provided we relax first to free our mind from its need to be practical and from the restrictions of our everyday emotions.

A visualised situation is one that has appropriate images. You can only visualise something concrete, something that you can feel, make a picture of, or point to. If an idea is abstract, nothing much can happen because the body cannot be provoked by abstract concepts. The emotional mind thinks only in terms of practical words and images: these are concrete words and pictures that the body can use in action.

The nervous system, on receiving such instructions, must first transform these into body code before passing them on. Its coding department will be stumped by abstract concepts because they have nothing to do with direct action.

To say: 'I have no pain', for example, has little effect: how can I draw a picture of I and having no pain? This I is an abstract concept that we cannot draw or point to: indicate your ego and you only point to your body. Also, no pain is a so-called negative idea, an abstract concept that our nervous system cannot put into appropriate body code. We can't draw a picture of no pain.

To be effective, we visualise ourselves with a more comfortable sensation. My ankle feels comfortably numb is a positive message that we can easily call up in our mind's eye, and our nervous system can transform this message into instructions for the body systems, and replace the sensation of pain with a comfortable sense of numbness.

We may simplify this as follows: imagine that your body has the understanding of a two year old child. We now reduce our emotional mind to this lower level of sophistication; the lower the level, the closer it gets to the body. A two year old only has to imagine itself vomiting to do just that. Young children may not yet understand the difficult abstract concept of don't do so; it is useless telling them not to do something. Tell them to stop.

It is only our emotional mind that can perform this creative job of visualising, not the rational-intellectual mind. Our rational mind is a builder. It must construct a situation or an image, and it does that in its own schematic way. This rational picture is like a pencil drawing if we compare it to the life-like technicolor image that is spontaneously evoked by our emotional mind.

Our rational mind constructs the schematic image in the same manner in which it re-constructs a memory situation. What did you have for dinner last night? Let me see, what was I doing last night . . . oh, yes, I was at a restaurant, and we had pasta and salad.

This is not the same memory of a past situation or event that is called up by the emotional mind, which is a re-cognition, a re-presentation, a making present again, a re-perception, of it. The process of visualisation is not entirely voluntary, and we should understand this clearly.

As children, we had little control over our emotional fantasy: we may remember the times that we scared ourselves by dreaming up frightening images, that we then could not get rid of. Children have such a vivid creative imagination that they may run crying from the bedroom. They created a monster in there that they did not even want to evoke, but they could not help doing it.

Adults have learned to exert control over their daydreams that young children do not yet have. They have as little say over the nature and direction of their day dreams as we adults have over our nocturnal dreams. Without outside help, children may not be able to get rid of the phantom that is as real to them as the monster from outer space is to us during our nightmare.

During stress, adults may worry and panic for the same reason. Like children, they bring up frightening images in spite of themselves. These involuntary images are under the control of strong emotions, so the rational mind remains a helpless spectator while all this is happening.

It is our emotional mind that indulges in such visualisation, and it may be driven by bad or good feelings. It usually works involuntarily, but we have more control over it when we relax first. We can set the tone (atmosphere) and indicate the initial direction by deliberately using appropriate words, and keep nudging it back when it strays or threatens to become negative in quality. We let our emotional mind do the work of visualising, and set the rational mind to watch over it.

Examples:

Sit or lie comfortably, and then relax with a few long breaths out, and by going limp all over, particularly in the face, neck and shoulders, arms, and legs. When you feel comfortable, then close your eyes and imagine:

(a) You are in your pleasant garden. Now establish this garden by looking around you and seeing the trees and flowers and other natural occupants of this garden: describe the scene to yourself. Then tell yourself a little story about a ripe, fragrant and juicy lemon you see on the lemon tree. It looks so inviting that you pluck it and then bite into it, so that you can feel its tart juice running into your mouth, making it water.

Could you feel some saliva flowing under the tongue? If not, go back to that garden and intensify your imagination: make the pictures more vivid by concentrating better! Practise this, if necessary, until it becomes effective.

(b) You are on the beach. It is a beautiful and drowsy day. The beach is clean, and is quiet and restful because there are very few people around. The sea creates calm and gentle waves, and you can see and hear their gentle restful rhythm. You are lying back comfortably on a beach chair and you can hear the gentle waves, the sounds of sea gulls, and the distant sounds of children playing. You now feel comfortably warm and drowsy and completely at ease.

When you read this story slowly while sitting comfortably, it should be suggestive enough to feel a little less tense, even calm. It should set your creative mind to work if you allow yourself to drift along with the meaning of the words: a sense of calm repose on a quiet and pleasant beach.

Play the game like children play a fun game: go all the way with the chosen suggestions and self-suggestions, exaggerate like they do, which is why they are so good at such emotional visualisation games. If you did not feel anything, go back to it, read it slowly to absorb the words better, and with all the enthusiasm that you can bring up: be like a child. Visualisation is child's play.

Having done this, and still comfortably relaxed, now create a pleasant beach situation by self-suggestion. You initiate this story by telling it to yourself, first with words if necessary, then gradually changing to images. It can happen that unpleasant things come into the story, created by an uneasy emotional mind. Someone may scuff sand in your face, or the sky darkens, and it begins to rain. Your rational mind keeps watch and intervenes. Stop, and go back to the pleasant setting, and then continue this good part. After a while, you will find yourself warm and relaxed, as if you had actually been there for a while.

Instead of the beach, you may, of course, choose any kind of surrounding that appeals to you, as long as it is appropriate to the effect that you want, such as a quiet and very restful garden setting to make you feel calm.

Remember that you deactivate your action system by visualising a calm situation, so that you must re-activate it for action, when you have finished. You do this by stretching and yawning, the same method with which you make your body fit again for activity, and your mind action-geared, every morning on waking up.

If I suffer from the heat and cannot cool down, I may relax and visualise myself swimming in a cool mountain stream. This will produce gooseflesh in spite of the heat around me. If, on the other hand, I waste time resenting the heat, the resenting process will be an equally effective visualisation of discomfort. I become more uncomfortable.

Resent discomfort and you double it. Relax instead and you halve it, particularly if you perform positive visualisation. We visualise ourselves in an appropriate situation for effect.

If I visualise myself as an invalid, I cannot expect to feel fit and fresh after such a practice session. If I should carry this negative image around in me all the time, then I perform consistent negative visualisation. No wonder I feel unfit and unwell. We are born pessimists, and it takes some courage and determination to feel well.

Our fantasy life, for this reason, may have a marked effect on our moods. Negative fantasies (of rejection, bitterness, or of suffering) before going to sleep may produce restless or even bad dreams, and depressive feelings on waking up. The reverse is equally true, but it seems to be easier for many people to be negative than to be positive in their fantasies. It takes a certain amount of faith and courage to be positive.

The visualisation sequence is as follows:

(a) First state what you want to happen in plain words that can be translated into pictures.

(b) Now let your emotional mind visualise the pictures. Do not try to construct them with your rational mind, because this only makes you tense up. Concentrate on the idea. Describe the setting to yourself, and just leave it to the highly creative emotional mind to bring them up like dream images, if it is so inclined.

The words visualisation and imagery are a little confusing here, because they refer to vision. It does not have to be a picture, however, it can be any form of inner perception: a thought, a feeling of texture or movement, or an inner voice that tells a story.

We can only judge this visualisation by its effect. If we can experience the effect, it is the proper mental image.

Concentrate on this job and do it wholeheartedly. These images must be visualised as intensely as possible; such concentrated attention pushes them through into the body, as it were. We should also remember that facility comes with practice. You can't learn to play the piano without proper practice. Your mind and fingers have to learn to adapt to the instrument.

The basic instruction is clear; if you find yourself in some kind of mess (an emotional trap or illness), visualise your way out of it. You do this by visualising the story of how you succeeded in doing this. In the case of infections (including cancer) you must correct what your body failed to do, and that is to reject the presence of these invaders in no uncertain terms. Whatever the terms you choose to use, let there be no mistake about the nature and strength of your feelings in the matter. Be as wholehearted in the creation of rejecting images as you can.

The visualised messages are decoded by our nervous system and appropriately coded for the body. Such body-coded messages filter all the way down to the lowest levels of regulation. Our job is only to provide the nervous system with appropriate emotional messages. How these are coded into actual body code is not our concern; the nervous system looks after that. What we say and visualise with great intensity is transformed into corresponding feelings, and these will then be coded into instructions for the body systems.

This process of self-influence is also known as *autoplastic* (self-changing) influence, and such self-influence works for involuntary negative visualisation as well as for voluntary positive performance. There is no need to know anything about anatomy. When I have the emotional intention (a want or need) to get up and make myself a drink, I don't have to know which nervous buttons to push. It is all done for me by my nervous system, as I perform the act of getting up.

If this is a rational thought instead of a practical intention then it contains no urge, no driving power, so that I can only speculate about the theoretical possibility of getting a drink. This is merely an interesting topic for thought, but no motive for action. To execute such a theoretical possibility, I have to suggest it to the emotional mind as a concrete want or need.

There are no hard and fast rules for visualisation. It is a natural process, after all, very much like child's play. If you can dream and daydream, then you can visualise. It is the same creative process at work, while you rest. When we begin to visualise, we must do it with all the concentration that we can rouse. We refer to this full concentration when we say we do something wholeheartedly, with all our heart, from the bottom of our heart.

For the emotional mind this means that we should visualise the topic passionately, with total dedication and devotion. This will involve a degree of arousal, but that is all right, as long as we keep our body limp and motionless.

If you visualise, then put your whole heart in it. Don't do it half-heartedly, like reciting a prayer while thinking of other things. It must not become such an empty routine. Visualisation is not an intellectual affair, and it is not an abstract architect's plan that you visualise. It is an affair of the emotional mind, a passionate affair. After all, it is your recovery that is at stake here. Practise it with all the passion you are capable of. The feeling of rejecting the invader, for example, should come from the bottom of your heart and from the marrow of your bones. Embrace healing as passionately as you would the love of your life.

To get into the visualisation mode, we must first relax our body, so we can turn our mind to the task of visualising what we want. Then we set the proper tone (atmosphere) for it. After that, we continue with a little self-direction to get it started, and then we let the story tell itself as much as possible. In other words, dream it like a day dream, and only interfere with it to ensure it continues in the right direction.

What about the content of these images? The images should be adapted to one's personal mores and beliefs. A general rule is: keep it simple and make it strong, do it from your heart rather than from your head. The more primitive such an image is, the more effective it will generally prove to be. Don't be too sophisticated about those images of healing. If it goes against your grain, change the image. It is all right, even useful, to bring up considerable anger at the cancer. If you find that difficult, it may hide a problem that should be explored.

There are two ways we can sit or lie quite still, if we suffer from cancer:

(a) In a debilitating apathy because of demoralisation. We feel completely powerless to help ourselves. We feel helpless and hopeless. We have given up fighting, and submit helplessly to the disease. We are now suffering from an organismic depression, a severe emotional illness that is separate from the disease. This is the effect on Mr TCP of persistently negative and involuntary visualisation.

(b) In a healing mode in relaxation. Here, we feel in charge of ourselves, determined to heal. This is an effect of positive and voluntary practice of visualisation.

Mr TCP should use the following images:

• Visualise himself as capable rather than powerless.

• Visualise the situation based on the positive working model he has chosen, in which failing is not even an option.

This means that the possibility of the cancer killing him is rejected totally. As we have said, this need not clash with legal, financial, or other arrangements he wishes to make, in case he dies. We do these things as a matter of routine before we travel overseas in case the plane crashes, but that does not stop us from going, and from betting our life that nothing fatal happens.

Mr TCP must say a big and wholehearted no to the cancer; he must reject this cancer spectre totally, and visualise that. The 'I must die' voodoo must be changed into an 'I don't have to die: I am free not to die, and I shall not die' belief.

That must be practised until this belief is well-established in his mind, and the voodoo removed: and he may need competent professional help to support him in this effort. Once this is accomplished, he can then use the technique of relaxation and visualisation to support his body in its fight against the biological cancer.

He should do this with the same taken-for-granted enthusiasm with which anyone, who decides to get out of bed in the morning, bets that the day will turn out to be relatively safe and routine.

Our emotional mind works with feelings and beliefs, while our rational mind works with concepts and knowledge. We should keep beliefs and knowledge apart, because they have no influence in each other's fields. They belong to different modes of reality, each with its own peculiar kind of logic, so that they don't mix. The twain shall never meet, and if they appear to, then it is only because we, ourselves, confuse them, and thereby ourselves. What I know remains separate from my body unless I believe it. Knowledge is intellectual, while belief is passionate.

To visualise effectively, you should picture that which you believe in, or want to believe in, as vividly as you can. Don't worry if this is not a rational notion. It is a belief that is capable of transforming us, not any knowledge, because a belief is profound, it affects the entire organism, whereas knowledge is superficial and neutral. Our organism works with feelings. These are beliefs themselves.

The feeling of fear is the unspoken belief that we are in great danger, and we act effectively on it by running. This fear is a life-saving instruction for our organism. Living organisms run on emotional logic which is entirely indifferent to knowledge. Knowledge by itself is interesting, but does not urge me to run.

Only a feeling can do that. We would have to bind this knowledge to some feeling, if we want to activate and execute it. In other words, we will have to believe it!

A right belief is a proper instruction that has an organising influence, but a wrong belief is a disorganising instruction. Right or wrong, beliefs work. Hypnotic suggestions are beliefs that influence the organism in powerful ways, if that suggestion is accepted. An effective belief that is instilled in hypnosis, is nothing more than an accepted suggestion.

The most powerful of beliefs is that of death by voodoo. This is an intensely disorganising suggestion that is accepted as a belief. It is extreme in its dysregulating power, so that it dysregulates the organism completely, and death ensues.

We can use the same power to our advantage and we do it by visualising while in a state of relaxation. This is a form of self-hypnosis.

How do we produce a right belief if we do not already possess it? Wholeheartedly accept a suggestion, turning it instantly into a belief. If that does not happen immediately, we can turn a suggestion into a belief by practising it. We establish it as a positive belief by diligent visualisation.

Chapter Twenty-four

THE ART AND TECHNIQUE
OF VISUALISATION

Visualisation involves the use of sensory images to influence our body processes. These sensory images do not involve our practical outer sense organs, but the free inner sense organs, those that we also use in dreaming. These inner sense organs are our original organs of vision, hearing, touching, smelling and tasting, as it were, that have not yet become reduced to perceiving only a practical reality for the sake of survival.

What is the nature of visualisation? Visualisation is the art of evoking images while the body is relaxed. The images that we then call up are not those of our adult imagination. They are neither the images of our practical world, nor intellectual constructions. This is why we must rest. We must first free our emotional mind for the job.

Life is a creative stream that powers our organism in all its activities, from dreaming to searching for food. This creative activity can come out in three different forms:

(a) It may be manifested in its original, and most primitive, form as the spontaneous and involuntary images that come up in our dream and daydream. These strange images are not yet made practical, or subjected to rational logic. This, if you wish, is the reality of the unconscious, or subconscious, mind. It is neither unconscious nor subconscious, but only differently conscious. Its creative effort is not yet made practical, nor is it limited by rational logic.

(b) It may be channelled into practical images and feelings for action, useful images for survival.

(c) It may be restrained by rational logic into theoretical thoughts.

We have to rest from practical action in order to dream or to think rationally. We wake up from the dream to shift into a practical mode for action-thinking, or into a theoretical mode for rational, action-free, thinking.

To understand this, we must look at how we have learned to think. After birth, a baby undergoes a period of practicalisation: a training in becoming competent, capable of effective action, of managing to do whatever is needed to survive. This is a performance training that is, in principle, no different from that of athletes; it requires a healthy attitude of the emotional mind and a fit body.

The infant's sensory equipment and emotional mind, as well as its other systems, therefore undergo a training in becoming practical. The dreaming baby becomes a practical infant.

The now practical emotional mind gives its instructions to the body in the form of feelings, and we call this earliest (most primitive) form of thinking: *feeling-thinking*. We still practise this in our routine (unthinking or unverbalised) behaviour, that is thus guided by silent and anonymous emotions.

We speak of having hunches, of gut-feelings, for example. These intuitions are examples of feeling-thinking. We may feel dimly, but strongly, that something is so, even if we don't know exactly why. Feelings are for doing, and not for knowing.

When an infant is about six months old, it learns to think in visual images. This is *picture-thinking* or *visual thinking*. Feelings have developed here into more flexible and elaborate, more advanced, visual images. We still have this imagery. When someone asks us to think of a horse, we may have an immediate but fleeting picture of one. This is a full technicolour image before our intellectual mind blanks it out, while it thinks of the word horse, and tries to reconstruct a horse in abstract thinking, a theoretical and abstract image of a horse.

When we relax and simply wait patiently for the intended image to come by itself, it will eventually appear in full detail. We dream at night, and daydream when we are idle, but we are also guided by concrete practical visual thinking throughout many of our actions.

Children are strongly dominated by visual thinking, and their play is a rich visual pageant, in which there is no difference as yet between practical reality and fantasy. This ability is also called *eidetic* perception. There are children who have this so strongly, that they play with imaginary companions (as we adults call them). Some lucky people retain this ability as a photographic memory as they grow up into adults, while others become so preoccupied with verbal thinking, that this capacity for intense imagery remains largely unused in daily routine, and atrophies. The average adult only makes use of it in idle day dreaming and in nightly dreams.

It is not until the age of two or two and a half years, that the child begins to learn to think in words: *verbal thinking*. Verbal thought involves speech and hearing. The child begins thinking in word-language by thinking out loud. Later it learns to suppress its outer speech, so that thinking becomes inner speech. Thoughts are therefore silent voices.

With verbal thinking we have gone far beyond direct practical thinking in terms of feelings and pictures. Feelings are so close to action, that feeling is simply prolonged into doing. Visual images are less direct, while words are farthest away from immediate action. The more urgent the situation is, the more our emotional mind depends on feelings for direct effect. It is capable of using images and concrete language, but uses these only in less urgent situations, where a wait and see attitude is an option.

Thinking in word-language also allows us to think of abstract theoretical matters, of things, events, and situations that have no immediate practical value. We shift our attention away from the practical world, in order to enter a world of theoretical imagination, the domain of our rational mind, which has no duties towards survival action. With thinking in words, we have strayed from our original intimate relationship with our body, and have become mere acquaintances of each other.

We began with thinking in terms of feelings, then images, then words, and with words we have lost direct touch with the body. If we have a frightening feeling, we feel and are frightened. If we have a frightening image, we are also frightened, but it does not frighten us as much as a frightening feeling would. A feeling is more direct in its effect on our organism than a visual image, while a word is least direct; it is distant from our body.

When we use words, we can talk about the frightened feeling without necessarily having it. If we want to experience it, we would have to go back in our development: we must change the words into an appropriate image, and this image will call up the feeling.

Mental pictures stand close to feelings, while words usually remain neutrally distant from these.

Our emotional mind develops from feeling-thinking to visual-thinking to word-thinking. In feeling, mind and body are still fused, and in picture-thinking they are close, while in using words they are far apart from each other. This is why we can think of mind and body as separate things, like Descartes did, only by using words to think with. There is simply no way in which I can feel mind and body being apart.

If we want to visualise feeling good, we use this sequence from feeling to image to word. This, as Schultz pointed out, reverses our developmental direction. Say it in your mind, see it in your mind, then feel it. In this feeling, body and mind meet and fuse, as it were.

 (i) First we move from the words to the image: say it and then picture it: see what you say;

 (ii) Then we move from the visual image to the feeling. Call up the feeling by concentrating on it, feeling good. Feel what you see.

We may bypass the pictures if we are not visually inclined: we then simply think the words (feeling good), and concentrate on evoking the feeling of feeling good. It helps, of course, to recall a memory of such a feeling good situation, and to remember (in particular) what it felt like.

Make a mental picture of I feel good in words or in a visual image, then feel it. This method is the working model for your future.

The technique of positive visualisation is now an established psychological technique and is used by athletes, musicians, and other public performers who wish to perform to optimal ability. It is also extensively and quite effectively used in psychotherapy. It is interesting to realise that novelists, who must use words to appeal to their reader's feelings, use the formula: see what you say, and then describe it, quite extensively. Describing an imaginary scene is an exercise in visualisation.

There are two reasons for using relaxation and visualisation as a method to promote our recovery:

(a) Visualisation in relaxation is essentially a self-hypnotic method for achieving more than we can accomplish by a mere intellectual decision to do better. We gear the more powerful emotional mind to this job; instead of having a neutral and indifferent reason, we activate a powerfully effective motive.

Relaxation is necessary to release the emotional mind from its biological task of guiding the body in action. Freed from this original task, it can now be used for other purposes, such as visualisation of more effective defence and healing.

Let me illustrate this with an example: we would have to have some extraordinary objective reason to put our hand willingly and voluntarily into a fire. Would we be prepared to burn our hand badly for the sake of a scientific experiment?

Yet, almost any parent will jump without much hesitation into a raging fire to save their child. That is the difference between a rational reason and an emotional motive.

(b) Our emotional mind is first and foremost a survival-action orientated mind, a practical mind. It is a practical intellect that is harnessed to survival behaviour only during our normal waking hours.

Outside these working hours, the emotional mind is relieved from its practical tasks, and we may then experience its full and freely creative potential in our dreams and daydreams. This creative activity affects our body just as much as its restricted guiding activity does during our practical waking hours. We are affected in ways, however, that are no longer limited to the immediately practical.

In a dream, for example, we are confronted with the creative dreaming of an emotional mind that is no longer limited to being practical, and our dreams are masterpieces of creative fantasy. Their meaning extends far beyond practical affairs, and the sensitive dreamer often remembers having experienced feelings that are not part of our practical fund of feelings. When we say that some beautiful music 'transports us to a different reality', we mean that we are experiencing strange feelings that are not part of our practical everyday world.

An untroubled mind may freely indulge in the most enjoyable of creative fantasies. The troubled emotional mind, however, is no longer so free, and can only dream up repeated nightmarish situations. The more narrowed it is by its negative emotional preoccupations, the more it will be restricted to a monotonous repetition of the nightmare situation.

This so called repetition compulsion is the sign of a troubled mind that is no longer free to change the theme of the dream. This is seen in shell-shock and other acute traumatic injuries of the emotional mind, including Mr TCP, who has recurrent bad dreams.

The motive for this repetition compulsion is the poverty and unfreedom of a mind that can do no different, that is no longer free to vary its themes.

When we want to use this emotional mind in visualisation, we must first turn it away from its preoccupation with the needs and actions of a practical existence. We accomplish this by relaxing our body until it is immobile. We relax our body to free our mind both from its practical and negative emotional (stress-induced) restraints.

We allow this body to become limp and motionless so that it loses interest in the affairs of the outside world. This has the effect of disengaging our emotional mind from this sensory world in much the same way as falling asleep does.

In this relaxed state, this mind is now no longer hindered by any practical and negative emotional limitations, so that it can be used for purposes other than our ordinary daily needs to influence our body.

We possess a reserve capacity of potential influence over the body that is non-ordinary. The word extraordinary literally means: outside of the ordinary.

This is the extraordinary potential for influencing our body that we make use of in visualisation. We can call on this reserve capacity for a better performance of the functions of healing than we ordinarily need. We gain access to this reserve capacity through relaxation and visualisation.

Athletes (and public performers more generally) use positive visualisation techniques to achieve a better performance. They do it for the following considerations:

(i) to gain a stronger motivation to win;

(ii) to gain a boost in self-worth and self-confidence;

(iii) to use the reserve capacity to improve performance;

(iv) mental rehearsal of the most efficient performance until it can be imagined faultlessly.

When we use visualisation for recovery from some illness, we do it for the same reasons, and we apply visualisation in two directions:

(i) Defensive visualisation – resistance and defence against the invaders; (ii) Reparative visualisation – healing (repair and maintenance).

In other words, we organise our organism for the best possible performance. Negative thoughts, fears and beliefs can hamper our efficiency of performance. Imagine a cat about to jump from a wall to the roof a small distance away; the cat has no thought, image, or feeling of failure, and is totally concentrated on landing properly on the roof. It jumps smoothly and effectively on to the roof and succeeds in its intention.

We observe that jump and say: what a little cat can do I can do because I am bigger and better. On the verge of jumping, the thought pops into our mind: what if I miss? What if I fall and break a leg? This negative image produces an organisation of our muscle system that will work at cross-purposes to the preparation for the jump. We should now forget about jumping. If we still want to jump on to the roof, we must first learn to relax, and then visualise a faultless and polished performance and rehearse it, until the successful jump is clear and strong in our mind. Only then can we expect to succeed

Anyone can do this relaxed rehearsal for a better performance. Your recovery is also such an anticipated performance; it is a project for rehearsal in relaxation, and for this we make use of positive visualisation.

We must relax our body if we want to engage our emotional mind in visualisation. There is no need to relax deeply for it, once you have learned to relax. Five long and slow breaths out while you allow your body to become quite limp and motionless (to unhitch the emotional mind) will usually be sufficient.

It is understandable that you may complain about your fate and bad luck while you are feeling down, and that will do no harm. But don't keep it up for too long, because this will amount to a negative visualisation. This is negative mental training: don't practise it.

Feeling low or depressed is an intense but paralysing negative emotion that brings you into a hypnosis-like state, in which you then start rehearsing the complaint. Let me stress again that it is not harmful as long as it does not last too long, and does not happen all the time; don't practise it as a wrong working model.

By all means have your doubts if they are real questions, and express them. Check out their probability with your doctor. Take all the practical steps that are necessary to put your affairs in order, but do this only to relieve yourself of that responsibility and duty, so that you can now concentrate on getting on with the job of recovering from the infection.

WHAT SHOULD WE VISUALISE?

The principle of visualisation is this: if you harbour wrong guiding feelings, they should be changed. Feelings are like quicksilver, difficult to work with. We have to give them form and we do that by allowing them to become images, pictures that we can hold in our mind and change if necessary. Changing our body is slower than changing our mind, but it can be done with visualisation.

Realise however, that this is a typical learning process. We must repeat this liberating visualisation frequently and regularly if it is to become effective. There is no magic involved in this or, to put it differently, the magic lies in diligent rehearsal (practice).

Chapter Twenty-five

MORE ON THE ART AND
TECHNIQUE OF VISUALISATION

In the last chapter we discussed the need for visualising an appropriate situation for the change that we want to create. Let us now take a look at the way in which such change can be brought about.

It is necessary to prevent yourself from creating the wrong beliefs about your illness, but it is equally important to get rid of any beliefs that are already present. Bad myths that are already present and active in the mind will act as hindrances to healing. We must learn to deal with both, and we can prevent and eliminate wrong beliefs through relaxation and visualisation.

We must relax before we are fit for visualisation. Relaxation is the proper preparation for visualisation because it helps to concentrate our emotional mind on the job. We have already mentioned that relaxation frees this emotional mind from its preoccupation with practical matters in the practical world as well as reducing the strength of any negative emotional blocks.

Relaxation has two effects on our consciousness:

(a) We develop a different kind of attention. This is a passive attention that simply calls up whatever it focuses on, without interfering with it. Our ordinary waking attention is a practical attention that is always asking: what can I do with this thing that I am aware of? We can experience this interfering quality very clearly when we become conscious of our own breathing: its automatic pacing stops immediately, so that we must actively take over. With passive attention, we can observe our breathing without stopping its automatic pacing. This same uninvolved quality of our passive attention makes it possible to evoke a feeling by concentrating on it, without interfering with its creation. Relaxation allows us to develop an intense total concentration on the topic. Let go, said Heyer so beautifully, and you can turn inward, and the inward comes out to you (page 90).

(b) We shift into a different kind of awareness. We take leave of the practical world around us. That world contains only action-related (practical) possibilities and, by turning away from it, we lose the separation of reality into a practical outer reality and the inner realm of fantasy. These fuse back into the original undifferentiated world of our childhood. We should remember that this separation is not there in the world itself, but that we have to create it, and maintain it in our waking hours.

This separation begins to fade when it is dark, or when we are tired, ill, stressed or otherwise in poor health: we begin to doubt whether we are seeing things, we can't tell whether we are dealing with reality or imagination.

The more childlike or primitive we become in our visualisation, the more effective it will be. Good hypnotic subjects are good visualisers because of some childlike naive quality in their make-up; they accept suggestions quite easily, sometimes even too easily, because of this ability. When they have accepted it, they then go all the way with the suggestion, while others often keep worrying at it, doubting and questioning, so that they don't get on with the job.

The reality that we experience in relaxation is no longer our practical reality, nor does it have anything to do with the objective-theoretical reality of the rational mind. This is an emotionally primitive world, in which the distinctions between inner imagination and outer reality no longer apply.

These distinctions between the inner world of the mind and the outer world of the senses are separations that we have learned to make on only practical and theoretical grounds, so that they are no longer valid.

Reality and imagination have fused, and so has their effect on our organism. This reality is an undifferentiated *physiognomic* reality, but we don't have to remember this term. This fusion can be achieved by relaxation, or involuntarily by any strong emotion, but also in times of stress: by exhaustion, illness, or injury.

A number of strange perceptual experiences are not part of the dimension of practical sensory experience, yet they are real and belong in the primitive physiognomic world. In this primitive reality there is still no difference between what is practical or not.

The child, as we have said, must go through a learning period, in which it develops the ability to tell the difference between a practical reality and that of the imagination. It must then perform this separation and keep this up as long as it is awake. We do this every morning as we leave the dream world, and move back into our practical waking reality; when we are idle, tired, ill or when conditions are such that it makes perception difficult, this separation is more difficult to maintain, so that it begins to fade to some degree.

The inner world of the imagination now invades the practical outside world, so that we lose track of what is practically real and what is imagination. We now have trouble keeping them apart. We mistake a towel in the wind for a ghost, we seem to hear the doorbell go, and so on.

This primitive physiognomic world is a world where things happen that are not possible in our more limited practical waking reality. Remember that our practical everyday world is only a very limited version of reality, a world in which only the practical-for-action is possible. For example: one of Professor Schultz's experiments with hypnosis involved the production of a burn blister by telling a young man in a hypnotic state that a glowing hot coin was going to be placed on his hand, and that he would develop a burn blister from it. The coin that was used was an ordinary cold coin, yet the man developed the burn. This could never have happened in a practical reality, nor in a rational one. In these realities it is simply not possible that a cold coin can cause a burn.

Yet it did happen, because it was produced in a different mode of reality, in which the man 'saw' the burning hot coin with primitive emotional eyes, and developed the burn according to primitive emotional logic that is not practical. We could say that it was his entire organism that responded to the burning coin, and not just his eyes.

The practical emotional mind would have fully agreed with the rational mind that this burn could not, and should never, have happened.

The primitive emotional mind, however, has no idea of what is practically possible or theoretically permitted, and says: of course that can, will, and does, happen. It cannot happen in the world of physics, but it is possible in the world ruled by a still very primitive emotional logic. This is the primitive physiognomic world in which the rationally and practically impossible is very well possible.

All hypnotic and self-hypnotic effects are produced by a shift into this highly creative but primitive mode of reality. The relaxation process shifts us into a mode of consciousness that corresponds to it. This is a mode in which we have access to such non-ordinary changes through appropriate visualisation. These effects are then achieved by a process of total focusing on the topic.

It is not necessary to remember all this. It is mentioned only to explain that you need to relax beforehand to make your mind fit for proper visualisation, and not to worry about having to use images that must be possible from a logical point of view. Let your creative fantasy do the work.

One of the steps in autogenic training involves the creation of warmth in the arms and legs. This is begun by focusing the mind on the formula: My right (left) arm is quite warm. This is repeated several times as a thought or as an image, until the actual feeling of warmth regularly appears in the arm. This warmth is produced by a widening of the blood vessels under the skin as a response to this self-suggestion.

If we think of mind and body as separate substances, then this effect should not happen. How can a loose and idle thought ever affect the body in any way? How is it possible then that the self-suggestion of a warm arm evokes the feeling of warmth that can actually be measured? How can I possibly reach those muscles that ring the blood vessels, and widen them?

Yet, it does happen: the self-suggestion of warmth during relaxation produces a measurable warmth.

This effect has been called the ideo-motor effect, and it says that every intention (be it thought, idea or image) calls up a corresponding bodily change. The intention is the seed of the completed change that develops out of it. This is sometimes referred to as the thought being the parent of the deed, but it is better to regard the thought as the seed of the deed which still has to grow out into this full effect.

This intention is not some thing that arises separately from the rest of the body. It is itself already part of the body, but only the beginning, and not yet a completed change. The intention of a movement is only the start of one, and must still develop into a completed bodily change. With suitable instruments, this intention can be shown as an activity of the brain.

An intention will develop into an appropriate completed change if we concentrate on it to make sure it does become what it is intended to become, so that we do not change our mind or allow it to become distracted from its goal.

Another name for this effect is *ideoplasia* and this describes another aspect. It states that every mental image tends to become a perception, or that it becomes as effective as a perception in bringing about some effect. An image of danger will therefore produce the same effects as the perception of a danger situation, always provided that this image is not merely a pale and ineffective intellectual one. This image must be as vivid as a dream image. We experience a dream, we live through it with our whole being, and this dream experience is neither practical perception nor theoretical imagination.

We must produce passive images, and we do this best by freeing our creative mind through relaxing beforehand. This will involve our primitive physiognomic reality again. As we saw, we are not limited to practical perception to produce effects. The adult categories of either practical perception or imagination do not apply any more. This gives us a greater freedom to produce effects that are not ordinarily possible in our waking mode. The visualised image is vivid and differently real from practical perceptions, but it is real enough because it is effective, because it affects our body.

We can perform a simple experiment to convince ourselves of how this happens. This is the so-called pendulum experiment that is very useful for passive-concentration training.

Take a fairly large sewing needle or any other pointed object that can be attached to a string to make a plumb. Now draw a cross of thick lines on a piece of paper. Hold the string with both hands so that the plumb is suspended fairly still above the intersection. You may support your elbows on the table or not, as you please. It is important to hold yourself as still and relaxed as you can while you visualise (imagine) the bob moving clearly in one direction: up and down or across. If you relax your body (as we have described above) and hold the bob still, it will begin to move by itself in the intended direction.

The better you concentrate, and the more still you hold your body, the larger the swings will be. If it does not happen at once, practise it patiently until you develop the ability to make it swing. This movement may appear mysterious, but its explanation is straightforward. Notice the following:

(a) The point of the bob will accurately describe the quality of your concentration; if you have only half your mind on the job, while the other half is busy elsewhere, or afraid that it can't be done, very little happens. If you lose concentration, or if you worry that it is not possible, or that you can't do it, the point will be still or it makes movements in the wrong directions: the other half of your mind may now be working at cross purposes.

(b) How does it work? As we have said, we can have an influence over many body processes that we ordinarily make little or no use of, simply because we don't need to. By holding the body still, the intention to move the point in the right direction is translated into the necessary body code by the nervous system. Only those muscle fibres that are needed for making the up and down movement of the bob are now activated. These fine muscles are ordinarily beyond our voluntary control, but they are well within our reserve of influence. This visualised pendulum motion is an extremely efficient movement, and it is also the basis for moving in Tai Chi or in other martial arts.

The relaxed state helps to concentrate our whole mind on the job, so that we achieve a stable single-minded concentration on the task at hand, undisturbed by any other preoccupations.

The image that appears in visualisation is neither a practical sensory image, nor a product of idle fantasy. It is a reality. What this also means is that we must define reality here in a different way. Real is what affects our organism, what has the power to change it. It does not matter if this image goes against all rational or practical logic. If it is capable of provoking a response from our body, then this image is real, and the logic is wrong.

What is real for our rational mind is not necessarily real for our organism. The moons of Jupiter may exist for our rational mind, but this neutral fact does not interest and affect our organism in the least; it does not affect it in any way, and is not real in this sense. A dream monster, on the other hand, is neither practically nor theoretically real, yet it is organismically real, because it makes us break out in an absolute panic: it is differently real. In short: whatever brings bodily change is concretely real. If it affects you, it is real.

There is therefore a good reason not to intellectualise these visual images. Nor does it matter whether or not they are practically possible. We are working with a different reality.

Passive concentration sharpens the quality of our observation. Perceiving is usually limited to a practical observation that serves our survival; we only see what we need to see to stay alive. We use a different form of attention for this practical purpose, an active form that is associated with a readiness to act.

Passive concentration can focus on feelings and images that are not part of our normal action world. These phenomena may be present in our practical waking mode, but we don't become aware of them unless they become useful for action. Let us look at two examples of sharpening our observation:

(a) Sit comfortably in a chair and relax. Now close your eyes, and take careful note of what happens. By rights you should now experience a sense of visual disorientation, because you have given up your visual contact with the world that surrounds you. Your visual orientation in it is no longer required, and it is cancelled. After a while, you should lose track of your orientation inside the room.

(b) While still sitting comfortably, open your eyes, and look at your hand while you tense it up. You can feel its practical shape very clearly so that you have a sharp sense of where your hand and fingers are located. This makes good practical sense when you have to use them for practical activities.

Now relax, close your eyes, and become aware of the feeling of this same hand. What was so sharply defined is now lost; its outlines are blurred, the hand feels fuzzy. This is no longer a workable hand, it does not even feel like a hand any more, simply because we don't need it while we are motionless and without intention to act. We experience our formless body that is no longer a practical body, but it is still a real body.

Our relaxed state offers us a whole world of new sensations to experience, if we are willing to open ourselves up to these.

Chapter Twenty-six

VISUALISATION: THE THEORY

INTRODUCTION

In Chapters twenty-three to twenty-five we discussed our preparation for visualisation in relaxation. This preparation consists of deactivating our body to release the emotional mind from its practical guiding task. We stressed that visualisation for healing must be performed in an action-free and stress-free zone.

The next two chapters give us a wider vision on the theory and practice of visualisation. This chapter introduces more theory and chapter twenty-seven examines practical techniques.

I. THE NATURE OF IMAGERY

Imagery is a passive-creative activity of the mind. It is thinking which is more primitive than sophisticated thinking with words. It is found in early childhood, before we learned to think in abstract concepts. Children's thought and fantasy are at first involuntary functions and it is only later in childhood that they gain a measure of control over their mental activity. Sensitive children may become frightened by their own fantasies, particularly if these are stimulated by intense anger or anxiety.

Adults have more voluntary control over their thinking than over passive fantasy, because intellectual thinking is an active process in which thoughts are being constructed with a degree of effort (intellectual effort). Intellectual recall is an active re-construction of the past.

This active constructive form of thinking fades as we sit back and become passive in relaxation. We cease constructing and begin to experience passive thinking; we submit ourselves to imagery. Thoughts are now no longer actively produced by us and we lose our sense of control over this process. Thoughts come and go without active direction because they are emotion-driven. It is as if we have shifted gears from active steering to an automatic progress.

When thinking becomes passive, thoughts that come up will change both their nature and their meaning.

They change their nature: words fade and make place for images (pictures, sounds) and feelings.

They change their meaning: words lose their rational meaning. This is a public meaning we can all understand and discuss because they are dictionary meanings. We can look these up and they have the same meaning for everybody.

The rational meaning of words and images makes place for an emotional one. The theoretical meaning of a concept returns to its practical origin and if we continue to sit in passive relaxation, even these practical meanings must fade.

An emotion is a private experience, even if it has been given a public label for discussion. Our emotional language is thus a private language for which no common dictionary exists.

The stronger our emotions become, the more they force a return to a more primitive level of thinking. If we are busy, this becomes practical thinking, thinking for action. When we are idle, thoughts lose their practical quality and become free from all theoretical and practical restrictions.

The common meaning of words and images now becomes private and personal and can no longer be understood by someone else.

The meaning of our dream images is so private that this can only be understood by our dream self. It is lost to our waking self who tries to understand dream images in intellectual terms.

When we work, our thinking is active and practical, but whenever we rest, we let go of active thinking. We now allow ourselves to drift along with this passive and emotion-driven stream of picture-thinking. We shift mental gears and move into the different thinking mode of passive thinking with pictures and feelings. Such images and feelings have little value for practical living, because the normal practical and rational filters of our waking life have been removed from our thinking process. Our thoughts are no longer filtered and screened and can come up quite freely from their subconscious source.

In summary:

• During dreaming, our emotional mind is free to experience without practical restrictions.

• When we wake up and shift into our practical waking mode, this act will fit a practical filter on the emotional mind of the dream. Now only action-related feelings, thoughts, and memories can enter our waking consciousness.

• When we adopt an abstract attitude, we put a rational filter on top of the practical one. This active attitude allows us to construct thoughts by voluntary effort.

Our waking consciousness is more limited than that of the dream. In our waking life, the greater freedom of the dreaming mind is cut back to practical thinking, while our rational mind will be limited to thinking theoretically.

In dreaming, we have no control over the direction that the story takes, and we passively drift with the flow of images. The fantasy of young children is similar to the dream. Once it has begun, children may be helplessly carried along by it, unable to change the story line in bad places.

Adults have two languages. We have an objective language in common. This intellectual language is removed from practical involvement in the business of surviving. It is a language for thinking about life while standing back from it, the language of a spectator.

We also have a private emotional language in which we become players in the field. In using this language, we may mingle emotional words and images of seeing, hearing, feeling, and sensing. Our self-suggestions in relaxation are of this mixed emotional kind. On their way to the body, our self-directed verbal messages for healing will be condensed into appropriate pictures. These inner images, in turn, will be concentrated into corresponding feelings. Feelings are translated into the appropriate body code that directs internal body functions.

The emotional language for understanding is a mythopoeic language that produces dreams, jokes, myths, legends, fairy tales, ghost stories, and superstitions. It is a natural biological language that our body understands intuitively.

It is also the proper language for healing.

As the child grows up, we said in chapter twenty-four, it develops three forms of thinking: first feeling-thinking, then imagery, and lastly verbal thinking. Its thinking progresses from feelings to pictures, and from pictures to words.

The younger a child is, the more it is limited to thinking in pictures, feelings, and the language of the body functions. It is a psychosomatic totality in its actions, and the child only needs to imagine itself sick to start feeling ill.

No sooner pictured than done. When the child imagines itself being sick, this image amounts to a total belief. That is its natural psychosomatic magic. We could illustrate the distances from word, picture, and feeling to the body as follows:

Word ⟶ Picture ⟶Feeling = Body

An adult would have to translate the words 'I feel sick' into a picture of being sick, and that picture into a feeling of sickness, to get to the point of vomiting. In using words we have come a long way away from our earlier feelings. There is a natural distance between words and pictures that we must cross when we want to make use of imagery for healing. This separation exists between our emotional and rational modes of understanding the sensory world. Every child must successfully bridge this separation in its development into adulthood.

No such gap exists between pictures and feelings because of a closer relationship between them.

By becoming quite passive in relaxation, we leave the realm of words and pass back to the world of effective imagery. We thus return to earlier forms of thinking: from words to imagery and from pictures to feelings, and from feelings into biological functions.

Emotional thinking. Our emotional mind has the task of guiding our body in action. The language for this job is primarily the language of images and feelings. This is well suited to action because it is efficient, it is impressive and fast. Feelings are ultra-rapid and intensely convincing, and images are quick and suggestive, but words are too slow and neutral for direct action.

We can't afford to take time to explain to someone in so many words that he should move away from an oncoming car. We shout our warning, and it is the emotional shout that does the job.

Our emotional mind can only understand concrete words. These are words that can evoke images, like those used by good novelists. Such imaginative words have the power to stir us, to move us, in short, to affect us.

On its lowest level, our emotional mind is subservient to the body and it is fully occupied with minding this body. This is our primitive (earliest) mind, an instinctive mind that can only drive the body into the necessary directions of survival action. An instinctive mind is an entirely involuntary mind.

In human organisms (and possibly in higher animals) this mind develops to a more flexible emotional level of guidance. It is no longer bound to total selfless service to the body and it has gained a little freedom for itself. This mind can now play and use fantasy for pleasure. It has such freedom only when it is not occupied with guiding the body in action. In these idle moments it enjoys impractical day-dreaming for its own sake.

Because the emotional mind is no longer entirely involuntary, and may now spin fairy tales for pleasure, this freedom also makes it vulnerable to creating negative and harmful fantasies about itself. This is particularly true of children in their inability to control their imagination.

Selection of images. Before we select a word for actual use in healing visualisation, we should check it for usefulness: 'Can I make a picture of it?' and if so: 'Is it possible to feel it in imagination?' These two questions will rule out abstract concepts that are beyond the limited understanding of our body.

Visualised images, wrote Dr Heyer (page 84), are not merely useless fantasies; they are real because they work on us. They affect us and change us. Images, he continued (page 86), can be directly understood by the body but words still have to be changed back into the appropriate language for change.

Unconscious or primary process thinking, said Freud, is mainly picture-thinking. The unconscious or subconscious mind is our emotional mind that uses its own brand of logic. As long as this emotional mind is not stressed, it is a practical guide for survival. When it is stressed it can no longer do its normal guiding work. It is now abnormal, a mis-guiding mind that can now only create problems.

Stress disorganises our emotional mind and its practical logic changes into an abnormal logic, which is totally useless for our organism. In stress, our disorganised emotional mind does more harm than good, and this should be sufficient reason to avoid becoming stressed.

Wavelengths of understanding. The meaning of abstract terms is usually beyond the understanding of our emotional mind. This is normally limited to the understanding of practical matters that we need for biological survival. Emotional logic is a practical logic used by mother nature to insure survival.

A word may contain a theoretical meaning that a rational mind understands. Our emotional mind may give the same word a significance which was perhaps not intended by the speaker. Even if our rational mind finds nothing of particular importance in a word, we may be severely affected by our emotional understanding of it. My head may well be clear, but my stomach is in a knot.

There can be a considerable gap between what someone says and how we hear it. The more intense emotions are, the wider this gap of mutual understanding will be between people. If emotions are very strong, this separation becomes too large for proper communication.

To close the gap, two people must get on the same wavelength of understanding. Only then can they hope to understand each other properly.

They may both decide to adopt an abstract attitude and understand and communicate words in their common dictionary meaning. They can also decide to adopt a humorous frame of mind and readily find a joke in some word. They may change to a tragic attitude and find it depressing. When we share the same mental attitude, we can understand each other clearly.

Misunderstandings arise when we are not tuned into each other, and that can happen when a patient visits an oncologist. They may be on entirely different wavelengths of understanding with disastrous results for the patient.

Visualising our understanding and knowing it. Our rational mind has no need to go beyond the word for its understanding. It nods to indicate that it knows its objective meaning, and stops there, because it has no need to do anything about it. A rational meaning does not have to have consequences, it is not obliged to affect us and to provoke a response in the body.

Our emotional mind translates words that it understands into appropriate pictures. It understands a word only if it can be pictured. It sees the word and feels it. The feeling, in turn, alters a biological function in the body.

A good word leads to a lift in mood. A bad one feels like a heavy hand on the heart or a sinking feeling in the stomach. Many everyday (idiomatic) expressions point to our awareness (understanding) by feeling: 'This guy gives me the shits' is a striking way of expressing the effective meaning that this man has for the speaker. He is equivalent to a cramp in the bowel. He is felt that way and this experience is made public in word language.

The emotional mind does not know anything, it feels and sees what the world has to offer. Seeing can be done both with eyes and mind. The distinction between 'seeing' and 'imagining' is something we learn to make because, for the young child, it is still the same thing. The child must learn to differentiate between the imagined and seen reality to become an adult.

Children still have a full capacity for visualisation, and we try to regain that facility. We try 'to be like a child' when we visualise; the distinction between imagination and reality fades away while our images become more vivid and convincing.

The difference between an imagined and perceived reality is a learned distinction that we make on practical grounds. Seeing, we then say, is believing, while imagination is not a true reality, only a fantasised one. As children, we painfully learned not to act on our vivid imagination, because we were ridiculed for that mistake. How often does a child hear: 'Stop that silly nonsense, you are just imagining it'. The child learns to devalue its imagery and loses its facility for vivid imagining through disuse. The word becomes more important than the image.

This distinction does not hold for feelings so that feeling is feeling. Feeling is always real, because we measure emotional reality by its effect on us. If it affects us, changes us, it is real.

A shift in meaning takes place. It is important to be aware of the shift in meaning that we mentioned earlier. Feelings, images, and words that we experience on an emotional level of understanding have a meaning that may be entirely different from their significance on a rational level. These two sets of logic and understanding can be at odds and if they are, our common sense becomes confused. It can't decide whether to believe the primitive emotional understanding of the stomach or the rational knowledge of the head. We have an emotional logic for direct living and a rational logic for knowing. Rational logic is used for thinking and for speculating about thinking.

The same sight, sound, touch, image or memory, has a different meaning in each kind of understanding. The examining touch of a doctor has an entirely different significance from a tender touch of a lover.

As we relax, we let go of our rational understanding and shift to the emotional mode of logic. On relaxing further, we even lose this practical understanding. We return to the free and impractical emotional fantasy of our dreams.

Visualised images that now rise up no longer need to keep their practical or theoretical (rational) meaning. Such images are not required to be real in the practical sense, they may not be part of our practical reality, yet they are effective. This gives us a greater freedom in effective visualisation. Our images don't have to be practically or objectively possible to heal.

If we want to influence the body, we can only do this through our emotional mind. Rational logic is ineffective. We return to a more primitive state of mind, and we achieve this best through relaxation. We abandon our rational-intellectual attitude towards reality and accept a different way of dealing with it.

A double loss of meaning takes place during relaxation, as we said. First we lose the rational-abstract meaning of the word, then its practical-emotional significance, and we are left with feelings and images that no longer remain hidden behind the screens of practicality and rationality. We change from using words to creating images, and for most people this means 'thinking in pictures'. Ernst Kretschmer, a noted professor of psychiatry of a previous generation, aptly called this process *Bildstreifendenken*, which means cartoon-strip-thinking (discussed by K. Betz in: *Handbuch der Neurosenlehre und Psychotherapie*, volume IV, page 143).

Words, pictures, and feelings are emotional instructions sent down to the body. Words are remote messages that may get lost. Pictures are nearby and arrive fairly quickly, while feelings are already inside the body; they have no distance to travel. Mind and body come together in feelings (sensations and emotions).

Of words, pictures, and feelings, the first to be created are complete feelings. This total feeling is the breeding ground from which pictures are born, and from these pictures sprout the words. Pictures only reveal part of the total-whole of feeling, and words can describe only part of the picture. One feeling is the mother of many pictures and one picture is the source of a great number of words.

Relaxation for effective visualisation. Before we visualise, we must relax for reasons that we mentioned. The method of 'relaxation followed by visualisation' is an ancient practice. In the West, it emerged from a marriage of hypnosis and psychoanalytic interpretation of material of dreams and of the unconscious in analysis. In the East, particularly in Tibet, it was practised systematically as part of the training of the mind for its liberation. This method has been applied quite effectively in the treatment of neuroses and psychosomatic disorders.

Therapeutic visualisation falls into one of two groups:

(1) The group of guided imagery. This was used effectively by the famous French psychiatrist Pierre Janet and worked out more systematically by H. Leuner and many others.

(2) The free fantasy group. This is unstructured visualisation and the procedure of free association in Freudian analysis is a typical example of it. You lie back (relaxed) and allow the thoughts, memories, and images, to come up without directing them in any way. What is brought up is then analysed for its meaning.

This therapeutic technique is aptly characterised as a 'waking dream' method. A waking dream state is a transitional state between involuntary dreaming and waking fantasy.

The first group is important for psychosomatic healing and we take a closer look at it.

II. THE NATURE OF THE WAKING DREAM STATE

Both our rational and emotional minds are conscious, but they are conscious in different ways, at times so different that it becomes confusing. Visualisation belongs to our emotional mode of awareness and understanding. We learn to ignore rational logic because it is a hindrance to effective visualisation.

Hanscarl Leuner made a systematic study of guided imagery and he pointed out that prior relaxation makes visualisation easier. This, in turn, deepens relaxation. Further relaxation facilitates the imaging process and gives our images a more vivid and convincing appearance (*Katathymes Bilderleben*, page 13).

We should give up trying to construct images by thinking them up deliberately, we abandon the active attitude of making them come up by trying with effort. We relax ourselves into a more passive state and let them arise spontaneously, just as we do when we drift off to sleep. We don't construct these images, we only need to correct them if necessary.

We shall experience – and this surprises many beginners – that by letting go of the idea of 'I have to make it happen', images come up spontaneously. We only need to become passive and patiently wait for them to come. A passive attitude will release our creative process from its practical shackles. A process of creative imagery begins that is neither dreaming nor waking, but a state of consciousness in its own right.

The stream of spontaneously creative imagery is an almost entirely involuntary flow. It is an underground stream that we are not usually aware of in our busy waking life. When we are awake, our attention is normally concentrated on the outer world because we are practical: we must live before we may dream.

In our idle moments, when we are no longer paying strict attention to the world around us, our attention will need to be less focused on practical matters. It slackens and we begin to experience the creation of spontaneous images. Thoughts and pictures drift freely in and out our field of awareness like projected slides. These images arise from a creative stream and they keep bubbling up into consciousness until we return to action. An active attitude restricts the freely creative flow to a practical trickle.

When we are busy, most of these creative images will be useless for the job at hand and they are blocked off from entering consciousness. Only what is relevant to the practical needs in the current situation is allowed through the screen of our attention. Our attention function has practical work to do and, by filtering out everything we don't need for the job at hand, it keeps our mind firmly focused on the present.

If this vitally important screening attention is disturbed, we could become so distracted from our present reality, that we could not function normally. Imagine how long an absent-minded person could survive in the jungle or on a busy road. Psychotic people have lost this ability to concentrate on the present. They have lost normal contact with the ongoing flow of the here and now and dwell in a disordered 'elsewhere'.

Relaxation lets us abandon the outside world, and this will allow the stream of inner images to come up to awareness. It is as if outer perceptions are replaced by inner images.

One explanation of this phenomenon is that inner images compensate for the loss of incoming outer (perceptual) images. A more useful explanation is that the attention filter has slackened its editing and screening work.

As we relax deeper, the quality of thinking changes. Words are replaced by images. These lose their practical and theoretical meaning and now carry an emotional message that is no longer geared to practical action. The same word or picture will have an entirely different meaning.

Our relaxed emotional mind is out of the driver's seat and free to roam the inner world. It creates images that express our emotional problems freely, unhindered by practical needs. They also express our emotional state better than words can ever do.

Professor Schultz, creator of Autogenic Training, studied the changing quality of our images as relaxation deepens.

(1) As we begin to relax, there are only formless images in the dark in front of our eyes. Greys and darks, with occasional strands of colour, come and go and shift about. We remain a passive observer of that activity.

(2) As relaxation deepens, we become increasingly passive and sink into a stage of visual thinking. We begin to experience a stream of formed images in front of our eyes, as if watching a slide show or film. We retain some direction over this stream and still recognise these images as ours.

(3) In the third stage, we lose our sense of familiarity with the images. They appear to be alien in character and we no longer recognise them as products of own thinking process. They are stable, and it can be disconcerting for a beginner to see an eye or a strange face in full detail staring back.

This third-stage imagery, commented Professor Schultz, is material straight out of the unconscious. (J. H. Schultz, in: *Der Weg des Autogenen Training*, page 35).

At this point, the emotional mind is creative without being limited to the familiar and practical. The images it produces are also the stuff that dreams are made of. Professor Schultz also brought up the interesting question whether such vivid and stable images can still be said to be mere images.

III. CLINICAL FORMS OF VISUALISATION

We mentioned the two types of visualisation in clinical use:

(1) Spontaneous or free visualisation. Here, you allow the process to run off by itself, without setting a specific task for it. This is interpretive visualisation.

(2) Guided visualisation. In this case, you are either given a specific situation to visualise by a therapist, or you set yourself that task. This method aims at diagnosing and correcting the emotional problem through direct visualisation, rather than through interpretation in analysis. This is corrective visualisation.

Visualisation for healing from cancer and other illnesses uses the second method. You are given a situation to visualise and to correct if it is wrong.

Guided imagery has been practised systematically by Leuner (*Katathymes Bilderleben*) and the name of his book states the essence of the process: 'Catathymic experience of images'. Catathymic means emotion-directed, and erleben refers to emotional (immediate) experience. You are guided through the experience of a series of symbolic situations that have therapeutic value. There is also a degree of interpretation involved in this system.

We shall discuss a form of guided visualisation which is practical and directly corrective, without going into symbol interpretation. This method was already applied by the eminent French psychiatrist Pierre Janet and references to his use of the method can be found in the excellent book on imagery by Mary M. Watkins (*Waking Dream*, page 36, quoted from Henri F. Ellenberger: *The Discovery of the Unconscious*, page 367) and also in Janet's two-volume *Psychological Healing*.

We shall find that this corrective method is in principle not much different from corrective treatment by hypnosis.

Examples of corrective visualisation.

In his book *Psychological Healing* (Volume I, pages 674 and onwards) Janet calls this method 'The transformation of a fixed idea (this simply means a conviction) by substitution'.

There may be traumatic scenes that are lived through over and over again in the subconscious life of our imagination and these represent wrong convictions which give rise to illness.

These memories must now be transformed, systematically and persistently, into non-traumatic scenes which can no longer do harm.

A traumatic memory is simply unfinished business. It is a story which took place in the past without losing its present character of being active. This current activity can only mean that it is not truly past. It is still present, still with us. The true past, said, Bergson, is our inactive history. If I can still wince about an embarrassing childhood memory, this still affects me in a concrete manner. It is still actual, alive and present.

If a traumatic memory bothers us, this story has not been taken to a satisfactory conclusion and here corrective guided imagery can be quite effective.

The task is clear: go back to that scene and finish the story. Return to it again and again until it has been corrected to your satisfaction. It is important to know that this may require repeated return visits because it is a myth that a bad memory can be erased in one sitting.

One could ask: how can I change the past? Am I not just kidding myself if I visualise a past event as having been brought to a satisfactory conclusion? Surely I can't change history? Of course we can't change history, and we are not trying to do that. We change the souvenir of this past that we still carry around with us. It is a current bad guiding image which influences our expectations, attitudes, and actual behaviour to an unacceptable degree. We only change our memory of the past, not the past itself.

A nurse, wrote Professor Janet, became affected by the sight of cholera patients and developed hysterical crises in which she lived through the fear that the 'cholera' would take her. In her abnormal imagery, the disease became personified into a frightening being. Professor Janet instructed her to transform this horrible appearance into that of a harmless clown. When she finally succeeded in doing so, she was rid of this nightmarish image.

In another instance a young woman became quite disturbed because her passionate love was not returned. She was obsessed with an image of her lover's face. Professor Janet encouraged her to question the truth of that 'beloved' quality, and to change the face into a beastly one. She did this successfully and was cured of her obsessive image, said Janet.

In both cases we see that the certainty (conviction or fixed idea) of the original image was expressed in its vivid nature.

This certainty must be brought into question, then transformed into its opposite, is Janet's advice to us.

What Professor Janet tells us here is important, and we may analyse this process into three separate sections.

252 You Don't Have to Die from Cancer

(1) We assure ourselves that we have the creative power to change a bad image. We shall refer to this as selfempowerment in the next chapter.

(2) We question the truth of our bad image. If cancer appears as a powerful enemy we query the validity of this belief and thus weaken our fear of it.

(3) We transform this suitably weakened harmful image into a harmless or destroyed opponent.

The difference between a good image and a bad picture is the difference between a positive guiding image and a negative one. Such images are subconscious guiding images. They affect us without our knowledge because they are emotional images. Mr TCP's harmful emotional mind fixed on dying is continuously guiding his body in that direction, yet he has no knowledge of it.

Guiding images instruct our organism in its behaviour and in its internal functions that follow outer behaviour. A negative guiding image may result in much harm. A good picture will be of practical benefit.

In bringing past unfinished business to a satisfactory conclusion, we have acted in an appropriate and efficient manner. We have guided the situation to its proper end by completing a practical emotion-driven behavioral ritual, and we have thus done with it. Coping with a situation means bringing it to a satisfactory conclusion. This is a natural ritual and if its completion is prevented we shall experience frustration in the form of anxiety, anger, depression, or guilt. When you feel an itch, the appropriate scratching act completes the ritual and ends the itch.

If guiding images are abnormal, they will bring failure and frustration into our lives, and frustration disorganises our health and well-being. We could now resort to abnormal attempts to bring the situation to a satisfactory close, but in vain. A frustrated situation is a failed one and therefore remains unfinished business.

To demonstrate the difference in the effect of good and bad guiding images, we take an example from a book by the Swiss professor of psychotherapy Medard Boss.

In an instructive introduction to one of his books on dreaming (translated as: "I dreamt last night . . .", page xi), Paul Stern tells us about a hypnotic dream experiment by Boss, who gave a number of women the hypnotic suggestion that they would dream about a sexual affair.

Three emotionally sound women reported without embarrassment a pleasurable dream. Two others, suffering from a neurosis, told a different story. One woman dreamt uneasily of a soldier with a hand-gun who approached her, and felt very frightened. The soldier's hand-gun, said Boss, is not merely a Freudian sexual symbol. It is the expression of a potentially dangerous encounter for this woman who could not imagine a sexual affair in any other way. Her neurosis limited her to an image of sex as harmful.

In this sexually enlightened age, commented Boss, a dreaming healthy woman should not need to disguise a penis as a hand-gun. There is no dream censor at work and the woman expressed her abnormal attitude to sex quite openly.

We may understand how this bad image of having sex could compel her to avoid it at all costs as a dangerous affair. The three women who openly enjoyed their sexual dream had no such limitations on their freedom to experience their sexuality. We also note how emotional logic works: what for psychoanalysis is a distorting censor, is merely a stressed, and therefore abnormal, emotional logic at work.

A guiding image may not be known (conscious as knowledge) but it is quite active in pushing us in a certain direction of behaviour. It may also prevent us from entering forbidden or dangerous areas of experience. A bad guiding image restricts our capacity to experience freely and to enjoy it without anxiety or anger. It may also prevent us from enjoying good health.

A young woman complained that she started a fight with her mother every time they met. She could not help it in spite of all efforts at self-control. During relaxation, I asked her to visualise her mother and she was horrified to see her mother with the face of a wolf. No need to wonder why they fought on contact. By gradually and repeatedly transforming this bad guiding image into a picture of a kindly mother, they got on much better. She was no longer mis-guided by the bad guiding image.

A patient reacted with panic to a suggested visit to an imaginary 'mysterious place where nothing is impossible'. Her panic ceased when I quickly guided her away from there to a calm and gentle country scene. That place was awful, she said, dark and threatening, closing in on her. This is how she actually experienced her world in panic, a world that is limited to only frightening possibilities.

By repeatedly going back, she gradually transformed that bad world into a nice place to live in, and coped better with her highly sensitive nature.

Another patient had a phobia for death in any situation that could in some way remind her of it (hospitals, surgeries, cemeteries). She felt compelled to avoid such places. In relaxed imagery, she saw death personified in a frightful, black-clad, evil witch. Following Professor Janet's example, I asked her to transform that terrifying image into one of a harmless and jolly clown. When she finally and consistently succeeded in doing this, she lost her death phobia.

A middle-aged lady had been unable to leave her house for more than twenty years. She has an obsessive personality and had developed severe agoraphobia. She could only visualise the outside world as a place of frightening possibilities, so threatening, that she experienced panic in just thinking of it. She simply could not imagine feeling safe out there, and what does this tell us? That 'feeling OK out there' was not a possibility that existed in her mind. She could not imagine the option of being at ease outside her house until we managed to change this wrong guiding image. By patiently creating doubt in her mind about the dangerous nature of the outside world, she very slowly (over some years) developed an alternative to the panic feeling, and to the image of herself as being helpless and giddy out there. 'Going outside' now became an option, a possibility that was simply not available before.

Persistent visualisation of herself 'going outside for a walk' became possible because relaxation reduced the giddy anxiety. This is one reason why relaxation prior to imagery is indispensable. She now walks long distances, and even ventures far beyond her suburb, and is slowly beginning to enjoy it.

A stressed business manager had been unable to sleep for some months and despaired of being able to sleep normally again. She hated having to take sleeping capsules. In guided imagery, she first experienced her bed as an enemy: 'I don't like the night and I hate my bed', she exclaimed. She then quite typically commented: 'It does not like me either, and won't allow me to sleep'. What was for her intellectual mind a bed, was for the emotional mind of this insomniac a living enemy with whom she would spend the night. How could she sleep in that hostile bed?

She was astounded to learn how negatively she felt about the bed, yet had no knowledge of it. Corrective visualisation was used to create a positive relationship with her bed, which brought relief. If such a bad guiding image persists in the subconscious mind of an insomniac, measures such as a warm bath, reading, and relaxing, can only fail.

Now an example from classical hypnosis. We take another look at Professor Schultz's burn blister experiment (mentioned in chapter twenty-five). A young man in hypnotic relaxation was told that a hot coin would be placed on the back of his hand and that he would develop a burn blister there in about six hours (which is the usual time for one to develop). The burn blister did indeed develop there at the appointed time.

Under exact experimental conditions in hypnosis, said Schultz, biological functions may be changed and returned to normal. All human functions can be influenced that way. The essential factor in this process, he wrote, is a direct and total concentration on the function that we want to change (*Hypnose-Technik*, page 45).

Let us now explore the meaning of such concentration.

The suggestion was made to the young man (and I translate):

'The coin is glowing [hot]; you won't feel any pain, but it will burn your skin'.

Hypnosis is a method for achieving total concentration on the suggestions of the hypnotist. As Schultz pointed out, every case of successful hypnosis is a self-hypnosis. The therapist is a convenient tool for use by the subject, who merely uses the therapist as a psychological lever for shifting himself or herself into a state of highly focused passive concentration.

From the point of view of the hypnotist, the burn blister should never have come up, because in his reality the coin had a normal temperature; it was not possible that it could cause a burn. From the point of view of the subject, however, the blister had to appear, because in this reality the coin was aglow, and he both saw and felt this burning coin. Even though it existed as an image in hypnotic imagery, the coin was real enough to have caused the burn.

What caused the burn was not the metal coin but the coin as an image that was visualised in such concentration, that there was no other option open to this man. He was convinced of the burn, and this absolute belief made the burn possible. He simply did not leave himself any other option.

This subject responded to the hypnotic suggestion with a total commitment to its meaning. That is just what passive concentration means. We now understand the self-destructive work that Mr TCP is committed to, if he receives a hypnotic instruction: 'You have three months, Mr TCP', this unfortunate man is dedicated to dying at the appointed time.

Could this burn experiment have been so successful with anybody? Only with good hypnotic subjects. These individuals have a natural talent for accepting such suggestions and for believing in them without question. A capacity for intense concentration and vivid imagery goes naturally with it.

Total concentration is total belief. It is impossible to be fully concentrated and still have doubts. A doubt represents a lapse of attention, a distraction from total focusing.

Let me explain this important point.

People can be arranged in a dimension from what one might call 'born acceptors' on one end to 'natural doubters' on the other. Most people will fall somewhere between these outermost personalities but we shall describe these extremes for greater clarity.

Doubters are thinkers rather than doers and their doubt often stops them from going over into action. Acceptors do before they think. For the acceptors the saying is typical: 'No sooner said than done'. They will jump in on naive faith where the over-careful and insecure doubter has no choice but to resist any suggestion of advance.

Acceptors don't look before they leap and they are often almost childlike in their trust of others. They are natural volunteers due to their low resistance against appeals, and swallow suggestions hook, line, and sinker. These persons are the natural victims of stage hypnotists, because they can't resist the call for volunteers, and they may already be in a self-induced hypnotic state as they climb onstage.

Acceptors are naive and suggestible, and naturally prone to believing in everything they have been told. They place an immediate and unquestioning faith in authoritarian figures.

Such personalities seem to lack resistance to outside influences. This natural suggestibility is a normal stage in early childhood, before the child learns to say I and No, and to resist stubbornly any suggestion that is not its own (H. Remplein: *Die*

Seelische Entwickelung des Menschen im Kindes-und Jugendalter, pages 241-2).

The doubter does not follow suggestions easily, and has objections which express an inborn ambivalence. You suggest one thing, and they will compulsively come out with the possibility of the opposite: what if it doesn't work, what if this, and what if that. They look and look before they leap, and see all kinds of reasons why they should not go ahead and jump. These are obsessive-compulsive personalities who are born doubters. They are ambivalent, indecisive, as if they have trouble making up their minds. Their doubting is not a healthy skepticism, however, it is a vacillation, which is an inability to decide on one clear way to go. Doubters are constitutional (born) fence-sitters. Such person-alities are not just careful, they are excessively careful because their ambivalence often makes them feel insecure and threatened.

The naivety of acceptors, on the other hand, gives them a strong childlike sense of security which is mostly lacking in doubters who feel eternally insecure. If the acceptor has trouble declining an invitation, the doubter has difficulty accepting it.

Acceptors are good hypnotic subjects because of their talent for believing. Their naive willingness to comply with suggestions stems from their facility in making other people's suggestions their own in an emotional strategy called participation or identification. Acceptors identify with the therapist and anything that comes from this person is easily accepted as a self-suggestion, because the difference between self and not-self is not marked out clearly enough.

The relaxing suggestion of a heavy arm is accepted easily and wholeheartedly. They may go all the way with that image and exaggerate like children: 'O-oh, I'm falling over on that side, that arm is sooo heavy.'

A doubter is unable to identify so easily with another person and finds it quite difficult to bridge the emotional distance between them. The doubter is willing, but can't make it: 'Arm heavy, hmmmm, let me check if it is really heavy . . .'. The arm is more likely to be light than heavy because of this doubting attitude which usually has a strong tendency to sway immediately towards the opposite of the suggestion.

A stressed doubter (assume a male) may not even be able to

258 You Don't Have to Die from Cancer

identify with himself, and is thus at odds with himself. When he tries to concentrate on a self-suggestion, he finds that he is unable to accept it and focus attention on it, as if it were an alien idea.

Most people have some of each of these personalities, and will entertain doubts about this and that, and have beliefs about other things.

When you wish to relax, work out doubts before proceeding with it. This is the right time for it. You should not do it during visualisation. This is the wrong time for it, for the same reason that a diver cannot afford to entertain doubts immediately before taking the plunge. Doubts now will distract from your full concentration on healing. Work them out before you relax, then abandon yourself with full self-consent to the relaxation and visualisation processes.

Let me summarise: believing is totally concentrating, nothing else. The burn blister experiment shows us that 'the magic of making it happen' lies in a total belief in the reality of the image and in a total focusing on that selected image. This intense focus can be likened to the concentration of light by a strong lens that burns the material it shines on.

What the acceptor-believer does naturally can be learned by the doubter, even if it has to be achieved by long effort and diligence. Learn to concentrate properly. Use the pendulum method, if necessary, to practise it.

Chapter Twenty-seven

VISUALISATION: THE PRACTICE

I. GENERAL VISUALISATION

We shall now concentrate on the method of guided imagery:

(1) To diagnose our emotional state.

(2) To correct this emotional state if necessary.

Example. We ask a stressed person, let us assume a woman, to visualise a landscape or a street scene, and she will probably bring up a bleak and threatening first picture, a scene from a bad dream. The mood of this image is one of profound unease or anxiety. With such a negative mood inevitably comes a feeling of insecurity and helplessness.

(1) Diagnostic use. This stressed woman may not be clearly aware of her abnormal outlook on life. Her poor frame of mind is present on a deeper emotional level that flows like an underground stream to guide behaviour. There are two reasons for this lack of knowledge:

(a) Emotions do not aim at becoming knowledge, but at provoking action. They compel our body without consulting us.

(b) We may be too busy to pay attention to the condition of our emotional life, too busy to stand still and take stock. Not now, we say, we haven't got time, we'll do that later, and we disregard those dim hunches that there is something wrong. We feel them but prefer not to know them. Just as we are already dehydrated before we become aware of being thirsty (thirst is too late to prevent it), we may be stressed before we know it.

A visualised bleak street scene or landscape is a direct expression of distress that threatens our well-being, if only we would stop to look, or remember the emotional tone of our dreams. This dreary scene often comes as a surprise: 'I never knew such a thing was in my mind'. The image is created out of feelings in the subconscious mind and gives us a direct view of what is going on in it.

(2) Corrective use. There is a two-way relationship between our inner attitudes and behaviour. Autogenic training is based on this free exchange: relax your body and put your mind at ease. Relax your inner attitude and your behaviour improves and vice versa. If you exchange a bad guiding image for a good one, that will also change your well-being.

The Reichian method of relaxing the tense body to ease the mind through massage and emotional expression is another example of this exchange principle. Body care improves the health of the mind and vice versa.

The principle of a two-way exchange can also be applied to corrective visualisation during hypnotic and self-guided relaxation. In the example of the visualised bleak scene, this person has two tasks. She must first take active charge of herself to overcome the feeling of helplessness that is always associated with a bad picture, and then take the initiative to correct it.

Leuner wrote that the first image in emotionally troubled people is often a bleak picture which improves in subsequent sessions. This is a common experience in visualisation, and to correct that image you begin with the guiding intention to do better. Your relaxed state makes such revision easier, because you can no longer feel stressed when you are relaxed. Your task is to revise the picture until it becomes a pleasing and satisfactory one, no matter how long it takes.

How do images relate to the emotions that accompany them? Felix Krueger, the founder of the genetic Ganzheit school of psychology, studied the development of psychological functions. He came to the conclusion that all thinking grew out of a total-whole (*Ganzheit*) of feeling, a mother feeling, as it were. This early feeling state differentiates into all later developed mental functions. We mentioned the mother-feelings of pleasure and frustration in the infant, out of which all later positive and negative feelings develop.

The feeling is therefore the creative source of the image and, later, of the emotional word. We must therefore first pay attention to the mood (general feeling-tone) of the visualised situation that is created in visualising or dreaming. Images that have grown out of it have the same feeling tone.

The feeling is the mother of the image, and it explains the meaning of that image. Our interpretation of that image must be consistent with the feeling atmosphere that gave rise to it. The image gives form to the feeling, it crystallises out from it like sugar crystals from a saturated syrup. A feeling becomes more tangible and conscious by taking form. We remember images better than formless feelings, because their form gives our mind something to hold and retain.

A panic reaction always begins with a mood of panic, and a delusion similarly begins with a delusional mood as its creative breeding ground. A nightmare always sprouts from a bad feeling as its creative source.

II. CANCER ORIENTATED VISUALISATION

Here also, we distinguish between diagnostic and corrective visualisation.

A. Diagnostic visualisation. What we want to diagnose here is how we feel in our emotional mind, below the intellectual surface, about the cancer in our body. The idea of 'cancer in our body' is a typical product of our rational-intellectual mind. Our emotional mind has no idea of what is 'inside the body', it can't think of cancer in that abstract manner. It is still primitive and, like a child, it personifies the cancer as a living thing outside the body.

We dream of 'things inside us' as being in the outside world, they become living entities outside the body. We even dream of our several selves in that way. This is precisely how the devil personifies the evil inside us.

We would dream of 'cancer in our body' as some foreign entity that threatens our life, and that is how we could visualise this internal danger. We visualise our relationship with this enemy as a confrontation.

Diagnostic visualisation therefore begins with a confrontation scene between ourselves and the cancer as our enemy. How do we see ourselves in the mirror of visualisation? Small, helpless, powerless? How do we experience our enemy, the monster that confronts us: large, aggressive, powerful?

A patient said that he had 'a strongly positive attitude' and was intellectually decided about that. His visualised image of the confrontation showed him up as a cowering little child facing a giant crab (cancer means crab), and he was shocked and disappointed to learn that he felt so powerless against it. He thought that he had a very positive attitude towards his illness, but he obviously felt differently about it.

B. Corrective visualisation. What should he do about such a negative subconscious image? He must correct it by replacing it with a positive picture. Before visualising anything else, however, he must first (to use a popular expression) empower himself. He must visualise himself strong enough to beat the enemy. Such self-boosting is more than a psychological ploy, it is part of our biological fighting ritual.

Many animals, when faced with an enemy, puff themselves up in various ways, so that they appear more imposing. This is done not merely to discourage the enemy but just as much to boost their own aggressive capacity. Warriors dance themselves into a trance, and then boast and hurl insults at their enemy before the actual battle begins. Verbally orientated people may talk themselves into becoming bigger and tougher.

We apply this self-boosting process in visualisation. If your picture is one in which you are the loser in confronting the enemy, you must empower yourself. Visualise yourselves being bigger and better, and the cancer being smaller and shrinking. Then, and only then, begin the battle. Rehearse this battle until it is clearly won, and keep practising your victory. Rid yourself of that harmful helplessness before you do battle. This is a corrective confrontation with the cancer. Don't be afraid of producing a possible negative picture, because that is merely the initial diagnosis of your emotional state of mind. Correct this into a satisfactory image that becomes your positive guiding image. This improved image will be a constant source of positive instructions from the emotional mind to the body.

It is surprising how quickly patients who mistakenly describe themselves as terminal, can respond to this positive guiding image. They regain their well-being by gaining weight and by looking better, and lose that false terminal quality.

The setting for a confrontation with the cancer enemy may be any situation that will serve as an arena. Let your fertile imagination also supply important supportive details, such as relatives and friends that cheer you on.

Any sense of helplessness in such imagined confrontations with cancer must be overcome, because it stems from a sense of incompetence in dealing with the problem. In a nightmare this helplessness represents the condition of total disorganisation of a being that is born to cope. Expressions such as I can't do it, it's too difficult for me, how can my mind change my body, are confessions of this disturbing powerlessness which evokes echos of the experience of helplessness of a totally dependent infant. A nightmare is a losing confrontation with a superior enemy. We experience utter helplessness in a hopeless conflict. We must never experience our confrontation with cancer in this incompetent manner.

The essential feature of a nightmare, wrote John E. Mack, is the dreamer's feeling of helplessness. A nightmare, he said, is the 'prototype of man's terror' and it describes a conflict with which the dreamer is unable to cope, and in which he experiences his total powerlessness. (preface, J. E. Mack: *Nightmares and Human Conflicts*).

III. VISUALISATION OF HEALING

Healing has since ancient times been associated with images of light and warmth and these are the images of victory over dark brooding forces. We switch on the light to dispel monsters and ghosts; daybreak chases away the demons and other evil spirits of the night. Light and warmth are useful images for healing.

We use corrective visualisation for healing. We visualise the normal state, over and over again, either as already present, or as being brought about by some means. Sending wave after wave of golden warmth into the affected area, and visualising that part returning to normal, is a good method. This has the advantage of producing visual images as well as the feeling of a healing warmth, which adds to the general feeling of well-being.

Healing baths are ancient images of healing that are also effective, especially where the problem is widespread, such as in cases of generalised eczema. If the problem (whatever it is) is more localised, it is still a good idea to begin with the imagery of general healing. Then follows a concentration on the affected area. This principle of 'treat the whole before the part' is a long tradition in medical treatment: improve general well-being before a local operation. The whole heals its ailing part.

A more systematic approach, using biological imagery, might

imitate the manner in which the body deals with an infection:
(1) A search and destroy operation, followed by:
(2) A repair operation.

When bacteria invade the body, say through a puncture of the skin, their presence is quickly detected and a fine net is thrown around them, so that they can't escape.

Captured bacteria at the site of invasion are coated with a substance that attracts killer cells. These leave the bloodstream in great numbers and make their way to the bacteria to destroy them. Blood vessels to the area of battle are opened wider as access roads to the scene of the battle.

On arrival, these soldiers can be seen to wriggle their way out of the finer blood vessels. They find the imprisoned bacteria, and the battle is on. It ends with the white blood cells digesting the invaders.

When the fight has been won, all fighting units move back into the widened blood vessels, and other white blood cells (scavenger cells) now arrive and begin a clean-up operation. This is followed by a thorough repair of the damage caused by the battle. That is the task of an engineer corps which restores the normal pre-battle order. It ends with a return of our sense of well-being: I feel well again.

If we add to this our personal effort to become as strong and fit as possible by self-boosting (rest, vitamins) before the battle, we have the following sequence for visualising:

1. A self-empowerment operation. Gearing up our emotional and physical fitness for the coming battle by visualising our position of superior strength in the confrontation with the enemy.
2. A search, locate, and trap the enemy, operation.
3. A destroy operation.
4. A clean-up and repair operation.
5. A restoration of well-being.

If you are confused about what and how you should visualise, imagine that you are explaining this confrontation and battle to a two year old. That should be a strongly visual tale that your body will understand. Put your whole heart in it, believe the story by vividly seeing (visualising) and feeling it. In total concentration seeing becomes believing, and feeling it makes it happen. We may question the word and doubt the image, but a feeling is convincing.

What believing is; believing is playing the game like a child. When a child plays it identifies fully with the role. A little girl plays: she is the queen, and her doll is a princess. Does the child really believe that the doll is a princess, and she a queen?

Early child psychologists spoke of role-play and make-believe, and claimed that the girl does not actually believe that the doll is a princess. In a little while, they reasoned, she will throw the doll in a corner, and if you ask why she so casually casts the princess aside like that, she will snort: 'That's a doll, silly, not a princess.'

They failed to understand that these are two entirely different situations. In the first, the doll was the princess, while in the second situation the game was over, and in this different situation the doll was a doll. In the first play situation, the child is convinced of the reality of the doll being a princess, simply because she cannot yet distinguish between being serious and play-acting. The child plays, but does not play-act, because only older children and adults can know the meaning of being serious and play-acting. (See also H. Remplein, same book, pages 236 to 239, and Heinz Werner, *Comparative Psychology of Mental Development*, pages 399-401.) The child plays for real and believes in her play.

This is the difference between a bad actor who play-acts, and a consummate one who totally identifies with the role, so that this actor becomes the role by believing in it. Identification and participation indicate a profound emotional involvement and this involvement is the identification of the good hypnotic subject with the suggestions of the therapist. Through this identification, the subject makes the suggestion his or her own.

The terms belief, wholehearted participation, total focusing, passive concentration, conviction, identification, are many different terms for the same process of full concentration.

Suggestions of healing and defence affect us through effective inner images. These pictures must be visualised as vividly as possible, they must be focused on with full concentration. That, in turn, means that these suggestions must be affirmed and believed.

The more vivid images are, the more they will resemble actual perception. We have faith in our perceptions. Seeing is believing, and feeling is certainty. In seeing some phenomenon in front of us, we believe in its existence, and when it now actually touches us, caresses or hurts us, we are convinced that it is real.

When we instruct our body in defence and healing, we must visualise these processes as vividly as possible. We should believe in our images, and we achieve that by fully focusing our attention on them. Full passive concentration is total identification, and that means total acceptance and belief, and successful visualisation is just that. Any doubt that we might have, at this stage, counts as a lapse of concentration.

Effective imagery. We spoke of effective images. What is an effective image? The glowing hot coin in Professor Schultz's experiment was an effective image. It worked because it was real and we define real as that which affects us.

A horrible monster from a nightmare is an effective image that provokes a panic reaction. It is real for our body because it works, even if it is not real for our rational mind.

Our body is, as we saw, that part of our mind which has taken on form. It relates to the mind as a picture relates to the total feeling that gave birth to it. The body is conscious on our most primitive level of awareness and understanding. An effective image is one that this conscious body can understand and we tailor our images to its level of understanding, which is that of a two year old child.

This effective image is a product of full concentration, of a wholehearted belief in the self-suggestion.

It wasn't the coin that produced the burn, but its effective image.

It wasn't the cancer that caused the psychogenic death, but its effective image.

IV. A POSITIVE ATTITUDE

This is a popular expression that is frequently used and often misunderstood. A positive mental attitude towards one's illness does not consist only of being cheerful and keeping busy, as if to show to everybody how good and positive one is about this. It is not only an intellectual decision to do well and that all is going to be well, because this will not prevent the emotional mind from sending negative instructions to the body. Intellectual decisions have little influence over the body, because the rational mind sits in the passenger's seat of our organism.

An effective frame of mind is an attitude of our emotional mind: it is an emotional attitude, not an intellectual one. A positive attitude is an effective emotional guiding image.

A proper positive attitude must be present in relaxed imagery, in which we take a peek into the subconscious mind (which is more appropriately called the emotional mind). This mind is the manager of the body.

What do we need for a positive attitude?

1. We visualise ourselves as competent and capable fighters, as confident winners. Confidence in the outcome of the battle is our working model and it is the directive that will be sent continuously to the body. An effective image of 'I can do it' must be present on the emotional-subconscious level if it is to work as an effective instruction. This is similar in effect to a hypnotic and post-hypnotic instruction.

The emotional mind must accept this positive image as a replacement for the negative one, and it will be the new effective guiding image. This acceptance by the emotional mind is an effective belief and we establish this by rehearsing it over and over again in regular practice.

A negative attitude of feeling small, helpless, powerless, and hopeless, is a hypnotic self-instruction for not healing, and a positive hypnotic self-instruction is a powerful motive for recovery.

2. We visualise our well-being. This is necessary for the same reason: it becomes a hypnotic self-instruction to the body. See and feel yourself well. We evoke a feeling in the same way that we bring up an image. We patiently concentrate on it until it comes.

A precautionary measure.

There is an important protective measure that must always be adopted during visualisation, especially if it is practised by sensitive persons. We must never underestimate the effect that imagery can have on the body, so that there must always be an escape route open in case one should feel helplessly trapped in some visualised situation.

We said that a visualised scene is not fully voluntary, and we might find that it can get out of hand. A child often experiences this fact in its uncontrolled fantasy. It cannot yet direct the story line and it keeps frightening itself with horrible images that it helplessly conjures up.

You must have an option for a self-rescue operation and that can consist of a magic wand, a helicopter, a spaceship, or any other method that allows you a quick exit from a bad spot.

Guided imagery sets scenes to be visualised, but it should initially be supervised by a competent therapist who knows how to deal with such crises and teach you that method.

Examples of potential traps in visualisation.

Asking someone who can't swim to imagine going into a deep pool may cause this person to panic and to experience drowning without being able to do anything about it.

An instant rescue is needed by an alert therapist to stop the panic.

Asking an asthmatic subject to take a deep breath in a garden (no matter how beautiful), may cause this person to wheeze if pollen or other plant material is a trigger for it. An instant change-over of the garden to a clean room with only filtered air, or an instant helicopter to take off into pure air, may be necessary.

Meeting a monster while feeling small and vulnerable may be as traumatic as a nightmare. The magic wand is useful in an emergency, because it can instantly change a bad situation into a good one.

SUGGESTION FOR A PRACTICE SCHEDULE

Here is a suggestion for a combined practice of relaxation and visualisation.

RELAXATION
1. Create the right setting and atmosphere.
2. Adopt a suitable position.
3. Unbrace your body.
4. Deactivate your action system.
Sharpen your concentration

VISUALISATION
1. Self-empowerment before confrontation
2. Defensive program
3. Restorative program
Cancelling
Practice schedule

Relaxation
Create the right setting and atmosphere.
Find a quiet place where you can remain undisturbed while you practise. Inform the family of what you are doing, so that they will respect your need for isolation.

Darken the room if possible, and close the doors against the intrusion of sound; natural sounds are not disturbing, but voices have a powerful attraction for our ears.

Make a short ritual of preparing yourself for the session, just as you prepare yourself ritually at night for sleep.

Adopt a suitable position.

Sit or lie as comfortably as you can. Undo any restricting clothing.

Lie or sit still with the elbows and knees slightly bent.

Close your eyes, and allow yourself to become completely limp and motionless.

Unbrace your body.

We brace against the day as soon as we wake up by adopting a defensive attitude, much like a boxer does. We draw up our shoulders towards the ears, pull the neck into the shoulders, and contort our face into a thinking grimace.

Undo this by unbracing: while you breathe out deeply (a long and slow sigh) unbrace the upper body as follows:

Lower the shoulders down towards the hips to unbrace them.

Lengthen the neck to straighten it and to loosen up its muscles.

Relax your face: smooth it out to undo the thinking spasms, particularly in the forehead and around the eyes. Drop your jaws to relax its muscles.

Deactivate your action system.

Relax your arms: just drop them. Abandon them, because you have no need for these operative tools for a while. Relax them by letting them become totally and utterly limp.

Relax your legs in the same way; they are tools for walking that you won't need for the time being.

Relax your face again: it needs extra attention.

Keep encouraging your face, arms, and legs to become as limp as possible for a while, until they begin to feel heavy, lazy, and fuzzy.

Sharpen your concentration on the tip of your tongue

Bring your attentive mind to the tip of the tongue.

Now keep it there by thinking rapidly: Tip of tongue . . . tip of tongue . . . and so on, until the mind has settled on it.

When you can stop thinking the sentence without losing contact with the feeling in the tip of the tongue, you are ready to visualise.

Visualisation

1. *Self-empowerment program*: a self-strengthening operation.
2. *Defensive program*: a radical cleansing operation.
   The detection of the invaders.
   The elimination of the invaders.
3. *Restorative program*: a complete repair operation.
   Healing the damage.
   Visualising full recovery.

What kind of images you use is up to you. Let yourself be guided by whatever spontaneous images come up. Remember that your emotional mind works with emotional logic; these images don't have to be rationally possible. In your waking mode, your body is a practical instrument, while in the dream this body is a habitat that you might experience as a country, house, or garden. Visualise as intensely as you can, and with as much conviction as you can manage to bring up to maximise concentration. If you can dream convincingly you can visualise effective images.

Cancelling

After every session, you must call your muscles back to work in the same way that you activate yourself every morning on waking up. Tense up to mobilise yourself for a waking day by stretching, yawning, and other rituals. Here, we use the following ritual that is used in autogenic training:

Take a deep breath.

Stretch your body, first gradually, then more briskly.

Open your eyes.

Practice schedule

Here is a suggestion for two different schedules. Select one or combine them if you have the time for it:

Three times daily for about thirty minutes.

Every two hours for ten minutes.

Practise systematically and painstakingly. Break it off if you feel bored or frustrated, rest for a while, and then come back to it. Don't do it with half a heart and mind. Devote yourself to it with a heart full of courage and a completely determined mind. It is better to do frequent but shorter sessions, than to practise one long one.

I wish you good practice.

Chapter Twenty-eight

QUESTIONS – PREDICTION AND TRUTH

With modern physics came the end of the concept of certainty because reality is now considered to be a chaotic process, one that is unpredictable and undetermined. Nothing is certain until the moment it actually happens. We cannot predict with enough certainty that it is going to happen before it actually does happen unless we claim to be able to see into the future. The old idea of certainty is now a statistical chance that may approach certainty, but can never reach it. It is now merely a probability.

Living phenomena are even more unpredictable, because we now have a chaotic process within a chaotic process and, of all living systems, the human being is the most unpredictable. We don't know with certainty what we are going to do until the very moment that we actually do it, because we are free to change our mind before that final moment. Our firm intention is all too easily distracted by unforeseen circumstances.

The human system is so complex, that prediction here becomes a frustrating occupation: we can rarely go further than saying: 'Chances are that . . .'

Any prediction about human beings has therefore to be taken with a grain of salt, even if it is based on statistics. Statistics only take into account a large mass of human beings and never personal-individual factors. Yet these factors constitute the unknown variable, and produce the individual variation from the average. We also assume, and perhaps too easily, that registration of statistical cases gives us an adequate picture of reality, if such personal factors are discounted.

The course of any disease can follow such an unpredictable pattern. The battle between disease factor and host regulation depends on so many variables, that prediction requires the greatest caution.

The course of cancer is no different; the same kind of tumour may grow faster in one person than in another. It can also spontaneously, without outside interference, grow or regress to different degrees in the same patient at different times. There is considerable variation in the interplay between virulence and host resistance. The cancer grows and shrinks, secondaries come and go, and we usually have no clear idea why all that happens.

What determines the factor of host resistance is a combination of constitutional (biological) and personal-emotional factors. What this means in practice is this: when you ask your doctor for a prognosis, bear in mind that he (or she) can merely give you an impersonal statistic, unless he (she) knows you well enough personally to include a professional guess about how you organism is going to deal with this.

Otherwise, what you are given in prediction cannot and does not apply to you individually, because it is nothing more than an educated guess in your unique single personal case. It is no more than a general direction that may, or may not, apply to your unique situation. Statistics can predict about people in general and never about you in particular.

What about our own expectations? Would we be kidding ourselves if we were to believe in our recovery? Is believing in our own recovery being unrealistic? Would it not be better just to accept the bad news, and try to enjoy what time we have left? We have discussed this attitude in the chapter on the working hypothesis. We don't know the future, and we can only work on a hypothesis of it: a good one or a bad one.

An attitude of accepting the cancer-death as inevitable, works for the cancer, and against you. The attitude of hoping for the best but being prepared for the worst also defaults to the wrong (non-recovery) working model. To accept disease or death goes against our deepest nature. We have a fundamental biological need to do everything possible to survive. This is a healthy urge that is not easily ignored. If it is not there, then we must ask: what is wrong?

As a working hypothesis, consider yourself in spontaneous remission. You have a job to do, and this is one that no-one else can do for you. You must become an active participant in your own healing, because that is an indispensable ingredient for it.

The future remains an undeclared and unforeseeable

phenomenon. No matter how unlikely recovery may seem from a rational point of view, this never means it is impossible.

Don't be misled by statements such as: spontaneous remissions are rare. They are not so rare. They go unrecognised when patients recover without going back for check-ups, and when they heal in spite of the chemotherapy, so that these numbers don't enter the statistics. People will buy Tatts tickets on the chance of winning. When can you know with absolute certainty that you have not drawn a lucky number? Only after the draw, and not before it.

The conventional saying is, as long as there is life, there is hope. This, as Dr Menninger remarked, is like saying that life keeps hope going. This should be reversed, he said: it is hope that keeps life going. Life itself is sustained by hope, and not the other way around: if there is hope, life goes on.

This is very important, because it shows that hope is not a vague spiritual thing; it is a biological factor, a necessary ingredient for the continuation of life. Take hope away, and life fades, because it cannot keep going without it. It was this kind of hope that kept many people alive, and against all odds, in concentration camps.

Hope is not an emotional luxury, it is a biological necessity. After describing four stages of psychological disintegration, Dr Menninger describes the fifth, and most serious, state of the mind, more serious than that of psychosis: the condition of demoralisation. Its clinical picture, he states, is that of a psychogenic death. There can be no question, he writes, that some people can be scared to death (*The Vital Balance*, pages 163 and 263).

Sometimes, Dr Menninger continues (page 386), hope fades and death comes, while at other times hope is maintained, and the impossible happens. This, he says, we know.

Hope should not be regarded as a consolation, not merely as an expression of sympathetic encouragement, warned Dr Menninger, because it is the expression of the life instinct itself in its fight against the forces of self-destruction (page 394).

The condition of demoralisation is a serious emotional illness that has nothing directly to do with the biological cancer but everything with the psychological cancer. This demoralisation syndrome is the experience of our own existential futility, a powerlessness to effect change, it is the helplessness and hopelessness of a completely trapped and isolated organism.

Mr TCP becomes isolated in his suffering because of his self-imposed death sentence, while his social circle contributes to this state of demoralisation and his eventual demise.

In cases of such psychogenic death, said Professor A. Jores, people die in the gaol of their own mind, they die in their hopelessness. He also remarks that doctors treat patients to prevent death, but do not help them to live (*Der Mensch und seine Krankheit*, page 109).

Their mind, said Professor J. Bastiaans of cancer patients, is an internal concentration camp, from which they urgently need to be liberated (*Isolement en bevrijding*, page 11). Hope is the liberating antidote for demoralisation.

Chapter Twenty-nine

QUESTIONS – THE TRUTH: IS IT HEALING OR DAMAGING?

Under the impression of being honest and frank, the telling of 'the truth about your condition' may often come out brutally. This telling of the truth may be telling the truth as I see it, or: telling the truth as my legal obligations force me to say it.

Even if, as the doctor sees it, this is as close to the truth as possible, it still raises the following questions:

(a) How near to the actual truth is this doctor's view?

(b) How should this statement be put: as an objective datum for entry into a computer file, or as a statement that is adapted to an emotionally highly vulnerable individual, who will react very strongly to the meaning that she or he may read into it?

The doctor cannot avoid responsibility by saying: 'I can only tell the truth, and how it is received is not my business'. The ancient Hippocratic oath, still current and valid, clearly states: first and foremost, do no harm. If the statement does unnecessary harm, then it is the wrong truth.

Dr G. R. Heyer writes (*Praktische Seelenheilkunde*): what is for the doctor knowledge and truth, is not always so for the patient. The thoughts that the patient entertains are not sober facts of knowledge, but feelings. These have positive or negative consequences on his or her biological processes. This is why, he continues, it is important not to harm the patient through a thoughtless and inappropriate scientific attitude.

It is not enough, says Heyer, to prevent the creation of such illness-provoking or healing-inhibiting images in a patient's mind during therapy, because the patient often arrives with these already present. We must uncover these wrong images and eliminate them (pages 12, 13).

Stated harshly, a statement that gives the worst possible outcome protects the doctor from legal complications. Modern medicine is, and should be, practised with one wary eye on the legal fraternity. The other eye, preoccupied with technique, however, is in danger of losing sight of the patient who is, after all, the reason for the existence of medicine, and the primary goal of all treatment.

The giving of an opinion, either by word or by body language, must be done in kindness, with due regard to the sensibilities of the patient. And the truth is always kinder than we think. This kinder truth is more in keeping with reality because of the following considerations: there exists a fundamental gap of uncertainty between the best of our knowledge and ability, and the capricious and chaotic reality that we live in. The French philosopher Henri Bergson, who had seen this so clearly, pointed out that it is to fill this gap of indetermination, that our emotional mind resorts to prayer, to sacrifice, and to other methods of invoking the goodwill of the gods that rule this capricious reality. Scientists try to cover this gap (in which anything at all is possible and anything may happen) with statistics, but these statistical figures are not the reality itself, but merely a quantitative attempt at an interpretation of a qualitative complexity.

This same gap exists between the best of our knowledge and the undecided future. The future is reality which is in the process of being made, and this becoming is not yet a reality (at least for us as organismic beings) until the very moment it is realised. Until then, it is merely a potential reality, unmade, incomplete, and undetermined.

The prediction: 'I know this to be' should therefore always be supplemented and complemented by the following: 'but this knowledge is never certainty'. There is always a fundamental gap of indetermination that is filled with hope, and that is the opening which leads out of the trap of inevitable death for Mr TCP.

One is therefore never fully justified in stating that death is inevitable. There are always exceptions that make a mockery out of such certainty. Patients have been sent home to die in peace, but these refused to die, in peace or otherwise, and prove that death is certain only at the ultimate end of life; it does not always follow medical opinion.

The ending of life is in the hands of the gods of chaos, who may issue a reprieve even at the last moment. And it is an important insight of psychosomatic medicine that the patient has considerable influence over this decision.

Accepting death as inevitable, and courageously and rationally adjusting oneself to this notion, may sound fine to writers of romance, but concrete organismic life is not like that. Close to execution time prisoners become apathetic rather than rational, and may experience altered states of consciousness as proof that they are anything but rationally resigned and calm. They shift into an altered mode that is perhaps nature's gentle way of protecting her children at the crucial time.

A problem may arise if members of the family want so called quality time with the patient. From their point of view, of course, this need for coming closer is understandable, even if the comment could be made that one should not wait for such an extreme opportunity for having quality time together. It also serves to ease the burden of an irrational guilt that so often appears in relatives.

From the point of view of the patient however, as we remarked in an earlier chapter, this could amount to bone-pointing, and could produce a considerable dent in her or his working model. Such quality time may have an adverse effect on the patient, if it is experienced as a subtle form of voodoo. Isn't it like saying: 'You are dying, so let's have some meaningful time together before it is too late'?

Chapter Thirty

QUESTIONS – HOW CAN THE MIND AFFECT THE BODY?

How can the mind be effective in bringing change to the body?
How can it influence our body functions for better or worse? For
the interested reader we offer the following.

We cannot understand how the emotional mind works on the
body if we do not see how they can interact at all. Our traditional
ideas about the nature of mind and body, and the way they can
interact, stem from the age of mechanics (seventeenth century),
and they are outdated. Let us take a closer look at these stale and
useless concepts, to see how they must be corrected.

Consider the words mind and body as we read them: the
separate words already make them seem like two separate entities.
If we say that mind and body live separate lives, then we must
explain how they can interact at all.

Our anatomy-based tradition wants us to say: 'the body and its
mind (the mind as the function of the body)', and then asks us to
look for this mind being somewhere in the body, perhaps in the
brain. We shall always search in vain, however.

Many theories have been invented to attempt to explain how
interaction can come about. The more clever they are
theoretically, the more useless they prove to be in practice.

The practical fact is that the body is in the mind, so that we say:
the mind and its body. This is how we experience the situation in
our practical living. We say that we make use of the body: I raised
my arm, and I braced my leg. This is the practical way in which
we experience our mind and body, as we live through our actions.

When we stop being busy and adopt an abstract attitude, then we
can distinguish mind and body on theoretical grounds, but no
longer according to practical criteria. The body is merely the
habitual activity of the mind, its relatively unvarying routine: this is
practical biological economy.

The seventeenth-century French philosopher Descartes (in the time of the scientific revolution), thought abstractly about the mind and body, and came to the following conclusion. The body, said he, is a material body because it takes up space, while the mind does not take up any space. And because it cannot be located anywhere in space, it has no substance.

He thought of mind and body as things in the same way in which we speak of thoughts, wishes, memories, and needs, as if they were things.

There are no such 'things' as thoughts and wishes, there is only the organism that thinks and wishes, remembers, imagines, and needs. We use such expressions for convenience, but we should remember that they are verbs, doings, and not nouns, not things.

This way of Descartes is an abstract, and impractical, way of defining the mind and body, because what he did was define the theoretical body as that which is not mind, and the equally theoretical mind as that which is not body. These are now mutually exclusive entities that, by their definition, cannot connect. What he defined as a body is not a concrete body, but only a thought about the body, and the same goes for the mind.

There is not much that we can do with such wrongly defined concepts of body and mind, because they are empty theoretical concepts. Their limited use as convenient working definitions is now being felt. A practical definition will be more useful to work with, and we now shall examine such a definition.

If we see the emotional mind as something that is originally separate from the body, there would be no reason for them to stay together, and because they are defined as being mutually exclusive, they can never interact. They only appear to be separate whenever we adopt a speculative (abstract) attitude in which we discern their theoretical differences and separate these into two different theoretical concepts. We can never make such a separation on practical grounds.

The emotional mind is not just a concept of the mind, and Descartes confused the workings of the emotional mind, which is a practical mind, with that of a rational mind, which is a theoretical mind. A theoretical mind can become very abstract and impractical in its musings, because there is a fundamental difference between a practical truth and a theoretical one.

The emotional mind is part of our organism, and we should say that it is quite substantial. This emotional mind is a guiding system that produces guiding feelings: instructions for the body to enact, to play them in action.

These feelings are not like single thoughts. If a thought is a sentence, then a feeling is the summary of a complete story. Imagine a complete film that is run off so fast that all we see is a flash of light on the screen. This is too fast for our rational mind, but our nervous system, that bio-computer, handles this information quite easily. A passing, fleeting, feeling contains a complete message for our action-geared body.

Feelings are the workings of our emotional mind in action, and they are complete instructions for practical behaviour, and for the normal internal regulation that supports such actions. When we have the intention to do something, to write a letter and to post it, for example, then this intention is a feeling that makes us do it. The initial intention and all other intentions to action are feelings. These push us into doing, they have a moving power, and this happens as follows:

The emotional mind computes these feelings on the basis of the needs of the situation, and sends them to the nervous system. The nervous system decodes and analyses these guiding feelings and changes them into appropriate instructions (body code) for the activities of organ systems and organs, all the way down to the level of activity in the cells. We may imagine that a mere intention develops into an entire system for action, in much the same way that an instruction from a director filters down to all levels of management, and finally to the worker force to implement it.

The emotional mind creates necessary instructions for action, and guides this action through; it sends instructions to the nervous system in the form of (usually anonymous) feelings that our rational mind may, or may not, notice. Whether it does, is not important for direct survival action, because the rational mind is too slow to be useful in emergencies. These instructions filter down to all lower levels of internal regulation.

Without such proper instructions, nothing can happen in the body, so that it is in neutral gear, merely idling. Practical instructions from the emotional mind put the body into gear. They prepare the body for action, initiate action, and follow it through to the (usually) successful end.

What we see passed down from the emotional mind to the cells is a free and flexible instruction that is gradually narrowed down to mere routine processes in the body. As the instruction filters down it loses in its range of options, and eventually becomes the only course of action left, and this is then executed. (What we describe here is an organic pattern of development, but we do not need to go into this in this book.)

The mind is the variable part of our organism, while the body is the fixed part, the (relatively) unchanging routine for action. We may change our mind, but changing our body is less easily done: we must rehearse this change regularly and often to make it come about. Mind and body do not differ in substance but in their capacity for variation, so that only by regular rehearsal can we form stable patterns.

Wrong instructions, if they are accompanied by very intense emotions, disorganise the body and play havoc with regulation. Such wrong instructions usually originate in emotional stress. The emotional mind is a practical guide to behaviour for only as long as it is not stressed. When it is distressed, it will produce instructions that are no longer practical, no longer useful for servicing and maintaining life.

Cancer is not caused by stress, but promoted by stress. It disorganises normal regulation (quality control, defence, healing, maintenance). Emotional stress is a 'cause' that acts on a different level of causation; the agents that can produce cancerous change in the cells during their division are causes on the lowest level, that of molecular interaction. Emotional stress, on the other hand, works its harm on the highest level of causation: that of the emotional mind. The entire organism is affected by its motives.

Nature's practical biological economy dictates that functions that have become constant and unvarying will be laid out as permanent forms, as functional patterns or as structures. A form is merely a channel, a fixed direction of change. Chronic harm will therefore become structural abnormality but, equally, chronic good will be converted into structural well-being.

An example. A cold virus enters a cell of the upper respiratory tract, and begins its disturbance there. This is a cause on the level of cells and molecules inside it.

When we ask why the child caught a cold, we are now no longer talking about a cell being invaded by a virus. We are pointing to the reasons or motives for a reduced resistance to the cold as an illness of the entire organism, which plays host to the invader. This motive acts on the level of the emotional mind, and that involves the activity of the complete organism.

Stress, working on the level of the emotional mind, may allow the beginning cancer to grow into the complication of cancer, that we know as clinical cancer.

Psychosomatic medicine is based on the unity of the organism. We may express this in a figure of speech by saying that mind and body are two sides of the very same coin. The word unity does not refer to a number here, to a numerical unity, but to a qualitative complexity.

It is better to say that the mind, which is expressed in the activity of the entire organism, contains the body, and that the body is merely the formed, structured, part of the mind.

In either case: (i) one cannot exist without the other; (ii) nor can one work without the other; (iii) one cannot work without influencing the other.

The mind, we could say, is the software for the body while the body is the hardware of the mind. Hard and soft, fixed routine and changeable instructions: there now is the real difference between body and mind.

This is a difference in degree of freedom to change and vary from moment to moment. The mind can change its intentions at any moment, while the body, as a structure, cannot do that. A nerve fibre can only direct impulses along the fibre, and no longer randomly. It is limited in its working to transmitting nervous impulses in one direction, and always in the same routine way. It is not free to do anything else, because it has a limiting structure. Body and mind merely differ in their degree of freedom of movement, and in no other way.

Look at your finger, for example. It has a special anatomical arrangement that allows the finger to bend for very practical purposes, for gripping. However, we may also realise that this anatomical structure at the same time limits this finger to this movement of bending, and that it prevents all other kinds of possible movements. All that freedom is lost, restrained by the anatomy of the finger. Our anatomical body restrains the mind to a practical function: it is the funnel of the mind.

The material that the body is made of is sensory material. It exists only for hands to feel it, eyes to see it, ears to hear it, and so on. This sensory material has absolutely nothing to do with the physical concept of matter. It only represents a restriction to having a practical form, and that amounts to a loss of freedom to vary. A structure is nothing but a fixed direction, a channel for limited change.

The rational mind should not be confused with the emotional

mind. It is occupied with thinking abstract thoughts, planning, and analysing, but has no direct influence over the body. It can do no more than bring up suggestions, and offer these to the emotional mind.

Our rational mind is even more changeable than the emotional mind. It is so free from bodily restrictions, that it can theorise, which means that it can think without immediate practical needs. This is something that the emotional mind can never do: it can think usefully only for immediate action. Our emotional mind thinks during action, whereas the rational mind must stop (action) to think.

The rational mind, because it is free from any need for direct action, can easily become impractical, whereas the emotional mind can only think practical thoughts. It can be forced into becoming impractical only by disorganising stress.

CONCENTRATION

The *extraordinary* feats that can be achieved in hypnosis or in any other altered state of consciousness (particularly in good hypnotic subjects), are rarely needed or useful in our *ordinary* practical daily life. We have no need for them except in unusual and extreme circumstances, and then only achieve these involuntarily, when we are forced by intense emotions into an intense state of concentration.

We have no need of such extraordinary performances in our normal daily routines, and we are never required to produce spontaneous bleeding from the palms of our hands in religious devotions, for example. Such feats are not part of our practical world, in the same way that dreams are not part of this practical waking reality: such phenomena belong to an impractical fringe of reality around it.

We do have access to this reserve capacity, however, and this is done through an intense concentration on the topic, so that one is totally focused on it. Such intense concentration can be achieved with relaxation, in which we select a topic and focus on it with this concentrated attention (visualisation). Relaxation calms the emotional mind by releasing it from its practical preoccupation with action. We can now make use of it for other purposes, such as visualisation. Visualisation is an intense concentration on an image, thought, or feeling. This is a versatile technique for improving our performance, and this performance may be the recovery from illness, or that of an athletic or artistic activity.

Chapter Thirty-one

A WIDER VIEW

This chapter may seem elaborate in a first reading, but it gives me the opportunity to provide a background for a complex subject. It goes into some detail to give a foundation to what has been written in the previous chapters, and it is aimed at those readers who are interested in some more information on this subject.

CANCER AND STRESS

We are witnessing a time of great upheaval in cancer research, particularly in the area of a possible relationship between stress and the onset and progression of cancer. There is still confusion about this relation, while there is much speculation about it, particularly where the lay public is concerned. There are some questions that should be answered if we want to be more clear about this.

Does stress cause the cancer? This is not a simple question that can be answered with yes or no, so that we must state the question differently. The reason is that there are different levels of possible causes, and these can be arranged in a hierarchy from the top level of the emotional mind to the lowest level of cells. This question, as such, mixes two incompatible levels of causation.

If the cause involves the emotional mind, we speak of a motive that provokes or promotes the appearance of an illness. We know from experience that stressed people become sick more easily, and that these illnesses tend to be more severe and to linger on: stress promotes illness by disorganising the body's defences. On the cellular level, we talk about physical causes that can lead to the appearance of disease, such as viruses, chemical pollutants, and genetic accidents. Let us therefore put the question in a different form:

(a) Can stress specifically cause cancer in the much same way in which a virus causes a viral infection in the body?

The answer is probably not, it is unlikely. There is quite a difference between causing cancer or a cold, and promoting or provoking it. These involve two different levels of causation.

(b) Can stress lead to cancer indirectly? The answer is yes, this is possible. Stress has a disorganising effect on the functions of the body, especially those that involve our regulation systems, and this disturbance can be profound:

● Stress may disorganise the laws that govern cell communities in the body; one of these concerns the control over number and quality in the process of cell division. We may compare this to those council regulations that control the building of new houses: where they can be built, and the minimum quality that these houses must have to pass the quality tests.

● Stress may interfere with our general and special protective functions against infections of all kinds. These defensive systems are made up of intelligence systems that report on any invasion of our body with foreign material, and of elimination teams to remove the invader. Cancer is no longer part of the normally regulated order of a healthy body, so that cancer cells may be regarded as invaders from inside. Cancer cells, coming from our own cells as their parents, are born delinquent, and they are traitors to our normally orderly system, which is organised for survival. They are infections from within. Stress interferes with efficient infection control.

Can a particular form of stress cause a specific kind of cancer? The answer is that such a direct relationship between specific forms of stress and cancer is very unlikely, because we would again be confusing two different levels of causation: that of the emotional mind and that of cells.

Can stress promote the growth of cancer once it has been created? The answer is yes. Stress is an immune suppressant. Stress, if severe enough, disorganises our body at all levels. It begins by disorganising the emotional mind, which failed to cope with it, and this disorder then filters all the way down to the level of cell control.

If a cold virus can cause a cold, must it always do so on exposure of the organism to the virus? The answer is no. Two conditions are necessary for the outbreak of the clinical picture

286 You Don't Have to Die from Cancer

that we call a cold and for its severity. This is true also for any other kind of invasion with foreign material such as cancer.

These two factors are: host resistance and invader virulence. We know much more about this invader virulence than about host resistance, because this invader virulence can be studied with physical methods, while host resistance involves personality factors. The personality is deeply involved in the ability of the organism to protect itself.

Three main factors blend to produce a negative influence on host resistance.

(a) A distressing situation (entrapment).
(b) A personal vulnerability.
(c) A local vulnerability.

We have discussed the nature of the entrapment situation. Now let us take a look at the two other factors.

Personal vulnerability. There is a certain personality that appears to be vulnerable to producing a psychosomatic disorder. Other types may predispose to neuroses and other forms of stress which involve a disturbance of the emotional life. In psychosomatic medicine it is the body that is the central player in the drama.

The word personality is merely a name for a practical individual coping style. We have made clear that the emotional mind is in charge of this coping style.

Every human being can become stressed, no matter what their personality type. Not everyone is vulnerable to the same extent, however, and the alexithymic personality is peculiarly vulnerable to psychosomatic disorders.

The emotional mind of such a personality is vulnerable and may fail to cope effectively with difficult situations. Its interaction is at risk of becoming sufficiently disturbed to produce a bodily disorder. If this disturbance is a long-term (chronic) one, the disorder at the front line shapes a path through the front-line system to the support system and lodges in some organ or organ system.

Characteristic of the alexithymic style is the peculiar lack of coping ability of the emotional mind. Everything happens as if its voice is too weak to come to awareness. The feelings it produces are not adequately expressed in speech, fantasy or dream, and this person is more aware of the body than of emotions.

The alexithymic personality closely resembles that described for the type C (cancer) personality, as the following shows. An impaired self-image leads to a sense of powerlessness and a strong need for conforming to social standards. There is an inability to get in touch with one's feelings, which are not recognised, perhaps denied, and therefore not easily expressed in speech, thought, fantasy or dream. (We may remember that the mother of the image and word is always a feeling.) This impaired contact with the life of feeling makes it difficult for such personalities to talk about their feelings, and they may even deny experiencing emotions. There is a remoteness from the life of feelings. Instead there is more concern with the condition of the body. The body becomes the front line with the world, it is the field in which conflicts are expressed. Because they don't have enough awareness of their feelings, they appear to have a rational-intellectual approach to life, and to lack aggressive emotions.

Local vulnerability. This is a weak spot in the organismic system that may originate as an inborn (congenital) weakness or is acquired through a previous illness. It can even be a particularly vulnerable moment in normal processing. The more complicated an organism is, the more prone it is to developing weak spots, where a local disorder can begin. We are familiar with the worn light globe that goes when we switch it on: the normal load of electricity is sufficient to break the wire in a weakened spot.

In medicine, such a weak spot is called a *locus minoris resistentiae:* an area of lowered resistance against disorder. Freud pointed to the use of a previously affected organ as the chosen seat of the new disorder (*Körperliches Entgegenkommen*). This is a halfway meeting of the body with the need to select an organ as the target for a psychosomatic disorder. The experience of a previous illness can also be utilised by the disturbance as a convenient ready channel to the target organ.

The three factors (distressing situation, vulnerable personality and vulnerable organ) work together to shape a path from disordered interaction through the organismic front-line and support systems to the vulnerable organ. This target organ receives the full force of the disturbance as a result of a failure of the regulating system to buffer it.

The blending of these three factors is responsible for the selection of the vulnerable individual and the vulnerable organ in this person as the seat of the disorder.

Vulnerability is not equally distributed in people. Not all people have an equal chance of getting sick. Illness in a population shows a pattern: some people are more consistently and more frequently affected than others and this is a common finding in general practice. In these clusters, illness does not occur at random but is related to times of crisis. As an additional factor to the weak spot, there is a faulty handling (personality factor) of such critical situations.

The term multifactorial causation is sometimes used in psychosomatic medicine to explain the complexity of factors that play a role in producing illness at the front line. The term simply means that a large number of ingredients are involved in cooking the local disorder. They blend to give the dish its special flavour.

A human organism has a certain way of dealing with the world, a personal coping style that is partly determined by constitution and partly shaped by learning. We may get by with the style we have been using since childhood until at an older age this is no longer effective for dealing with adult crisis situations. The result of this interaction between an inadequate personal coping style with a distressing situation leads to disorganisation at the front line. Disorganising instructions now leave the front line for the support system, only to throw it into equal chaos. A wave of disorder courses through the support system and finds a local weak spot, a vulnerable organ, as a target.

The old idea in psychosomatic medicine that specific conflicts lead to specific illnesses has now been abandoned.

The selective factor is not bound to specific problems and this makes it unlikely that cancer is specifically a product of bereavement and depression. Behind the insoluble conflict stands a vulnerable personality, and behind that a vulnerable support system (organ systems and organs).

The current upheaval in cancer research is a phenomenon that is common with any new development in science or medicine. Initially, the picture of this development is quite unclear and uncertain, but becomes more clearly focused as this new development goes on to more sophisticated and advanced methods of testing, and to better definitions of what it is that is being studied.

When stress is being studied, for example, we should ask: what is stress exactly? The answer often is: we don't know, but we define it as such and such, and we study that definition.

When we study the mind, what is this mind? What is attention? What is consciousness? What is an emotion? These concepts sound so familiar, that we are inclined to take them for granted. There is no precise answer to such questions and researchers can only give working definitions of the phenomenon. What is being studied in the experiment is not the original, but only a working definition of it. And if each researcher gives his or her own definition, we can become more confused.

At the moment there are three lines of cancer research:

Research into new forms of treatment: drug treatment and, more promising, a safer immune therapy.

Cancer therapy (chemotherapy and radiotherapy) aş it is now, is still a paradoxical form of treatment. Why?

(a) The idea behind chemotherapy is clear; cancer cells are biologically much weaker cells than the more sturdy normal tissue cells. If you introduce a carefully dosed cell poison into the system, this will kill mainly the weaker cancer cells. If we can find poisons that certain cancer cells are particularly sensitive to, so much the better. The more specific the poison is for the type of cancer cell, and the more it can spare the normal cell, the better it is.

(b) In practice, many of these drugs are still unspecific, and they can have potentially serious side-effects. They are, unfortunately, also immune-suppressants and, because of this effect, they may promote infections and other types of cancer to come up elsewhere in the body, either at the time of treatment, or even years later. Cancer cells may also develop a resistance to the drugs, like bacteria do to antibiotics.

This is why the practice of chemotherapy and radiotherapy has been called a double-edged sword. Some of these drugs are the same ones that are being used in organ transplantations, in order to cancel the immune system, which would otherwise have activated the body's elimination teams.

Chemotherapy itself is not a consistent form of treatment. There is an exact form of chemotherapy, in which a precise drug is available and indicated for a specific cancer. There is also a more experimental approach if this fails, or if there is no specific drug available, so that it becomes a matter of: 'Let's try this, and if that doesn't work let's try something else, and hope that it works'.

(c) The side-effects on the patient can be demoralising in their severity, in spite of counteracting drugs. Patients are often reluctant to complain about these side-effects, and their specialists may not have an adequate idea of the extent of their suffering.

The fear of chemotherapy and radiotherapy that many patients have and may not express, is therefore not unfounded. There is an additional problem with drug treatment that is related to the side effects. You prescribe one drug, and you may need to give another one to counter the side-effects of the first one, and sometimes a third drug to reduce the side-effects of the second one.

The fear: 'I may be prescribed more drugs, and I feel bad enough already', may prevent patients from speaking up. It is important to discuss these side-effects with your oncologist, however, because there may be new and effective counteracting drugs available.

Research into cancer prevention: this important area is now receiving more attention, because it has been effective in the past with many other forms of infection, such as tuberculosis, diphtheria, tetanus, smallpox, poliomyelitis, and so on.

Our diets and other living habits will have to be closely examined, and the environment will be more carefully studied for potential cancer-producing and cancer-promoting effects.

So far, research has concentrated on cancer in its biological form. Recently a new line of study was begun:

Research into the psychosomatic aspects of cancer. In spite of the attitude of some oncologists that psychological factors are not relevant, or at the most a side issue, there is now a growing amount of research being done in this field.

Brave souls began this controversial change in cancer research by daring to break through the body-mind barrier that was set up by the conservative tradition in medicine.

This was a tradition that was based on the classical-physical principles of science, and the materialist philosophy behind it. The material curtain between mind and body is kin to the late Iron Curtain in the days of the USSR. It is a barrier that says: 'Mind stay out. You have no influence here in this realm of Physical Matter'. In one of the strict materialist interpretations, the mind was reduced to being no more than a phosphorescence of the working brain, like the glow over a city at night. This conservative tradition is based on a naive confusion between the concept of physical matter, and the experience of sensory material, but we shall not go into that here.

The study of medicine began with the study of anatomy, which is the sensory structure of the body: that part which we can see and feel. Then came physiology, which studies the work that these anatomical structures do. It considers functions to be secondary to structures: structural functions. After that came pathology, which studies diseased structures. Then pathophysiology, that studies the abnormal functions of these diseased structures. Last and always least came psychology, which studied the mind, and nobody could say how this mind connected up with anatomy and physiology. For this reason, psychology always remained an uncomfortable – and barely welcome – outsider in the house of medicine.

Although psychosomatic medicine was reluctantly admitted as a member in the late 1930s, it has not been fully accepted by the believers in traditional materialism. Like any outsider, psychology could not enter into the current conversation about medical conditions of the body, and could not fit in comfortably. One of the reasons for this is that it regards functions as primary to structures, so that it asks what the structures are that are created by the functions.

This materialist approach can be compared to studying computer hardware without considering the effects of the software that is to run it (and that has been the motive for its creation in a self-creative organic system). The materialist approach is, therefore, that a function must emerge from a structure, and that it is therefore merely a part of this larger structure. Psychosomatic medicine reverses this situation: the function is the larger phenomenon, and the structure emerges from this function as merely its routine part. The function contains the structure, the mind contains the body as its habitual aspect.

MIND AND MATTER

The question that is being fought over is this: can (and does) stress play a significant role in the onset and development of cancer? This, of course, is another way of putting the basic question: can the mind, in its normal and abnormal condition, affect the body in its material functions and structures? And if so, how?

The answer to the first question is: yes, it can and does.

The reasoning behind this (which is too complicated to discuss more fully here) is that there is a fundamental difference between the material of the world around us that we experience with our sensory organs (this is all that we see, hear, feel, taste, and smell) and the theoretical concept of matter in the physical sciences (which is stuff that we can never actually experience, but can only think of).

Our body, the body that we see and feel, the body of muscles and blood and brain and bones, is an experienced body after all, a sensory body that we see, touch, and smell; it is made up of sensory material. It is also this sensory body that we are talking about, and if there is cancer in it, then this is also a sensory experience: it consists of sensory material. The emotional mind is in charge of this sensory experience, and of all our responses to it. Sensory material is the fixed, relatively unchanging, part of the organism, the stable part of sensory experience. The hardness and solidity of bone to our touch is its unchanging state, while the mind is formless and variable in our experience of it.

Freud described the strange effects that emotional distress can have on the functions of the body in certain personalities (so called hysterical personalities). There was no doubt about the relationship, but he could only speak of 'a mysterious leap from the mind to the body'.

In other words: the wrong emotion somehow invades the body and produces its effects there. That is what appears to happen but we don't know how an immaterial mind could jump the (physical) material barrier.

For example: A patient develops a paralysis of the legs, and cannot walk. The neurologist cannot find anything wrong with the legs. What he (assuming a male) is going to say now, will depend on whether he works from behind the material curtain.

If he works behind the curtain, he will say: 'There is nothing wrong with you, it's only your imagination'. What he means to say is that emotional troubles cannot be the cause of such a paralysis. He is also saying that the paralysis is therefore not real (because it is not structural), meaning: 'It's not really that you can't, you just think you can't, or maybe you just won't'.

If he has experience in psychosomatic medicine, he will say: 'I accept that you can't walk, but I cannot find any reason for that in your sensory body. The paralysis cannot be found in the legs, in its muscles and nerves, so that it must be located higher up, in the function centres that give the instructions to move the legs like tools, and that means: your practical emotional mind. This emotional mind is a guiding centre that is responsible for normal survival behaviour, and it gives practical instructions to the body about what to do in what situation. In your case there is an abnormal instruction not to walk. That region is no longer my field, so that you should see a psychotherapist.'

Psychosomatic medicine is a child of psychoanalysis, many say; this may be true in the US and England, but not in continental Europe, where it has two different parents: psychoanalysis and phenomenology.

What is phenomenology? It is the determination to find a better way of studying the relationship between mind and body, because the traditional idea has worked for a while, but is no longer useful. In fact, this old idea of body and mind as separate substances can only hamper further understanding. It has become stale and needs to be thrown out.

This need to change our basic concepts comes up all the time in research, and all progress is based on such change. In the physical sciences, Planck and Einstein revolutionised the basic tools of physical thinking, so that physics made a great leap forward in our century.

The outdated tool in medicine was born as an idea of the French philosopher Descartes, who said: what is matter? Never mind. What is mind? No matter. This was a witty comment, made later, on his theory that mind had no material substance, while the body was only material substance. There you have the material barrier: whatever is not made of physical matter is not real, only illusion or imagination.

It is, of course, nonsense that the mind is immaterial, it was only Descartes who thought that it was so.

Descartes made the concepts of body and mind into two totally different and independent things: he separated them, and we are still uselessly trying to undo the damage by bringing them together again. Philosophers and scientists have gone through contortions of thinking to try to fuse them, always in vain.

Phenomenology has shown that this is wrong. It cannot be done because body and mind are working definitions that are mutually exclusive. What is mind? All that is not body. What is body? All that is not mind. Each is actually defined by the absence of the other, so that it is useless to try to connect them. It was fitting that it was also a French philosopher who was capable of correcting the false ideas of Descartes. This was the brilliant Henri Bergson, who became a legend in his own lifetime, and who was a welcome fresh and cleansing breeze in the stale and musty world of thought.

Phenomenology has thrown these misguided concepts overboard, because they are based on wrong thinking, and useful only as working definitions. A new movement has appeared which has destroyed the material curtain, and the name of that movement is phenomenological psychology. Bergson, Buytendijk, van den Berg, von Weizsäcker, Straus, Schultz, and von Gebsattel, are a few of the important names behind the revolution in thinking about our living organism.

A USEFUL WAY OF LOOKING AT MIND AND BODY

The difference between mind and body has nothing to do with matter being present or not. It has to do with a difference in degree of possible variation, but this is not important here.

What is important is that the mind contains the body inside itself; the relatively fixed body is located in the variable mind, and always influenced by it. Our immediate experience is that our mind envelops our body, that this body is inside our organism. The thought that our mind must be located inside our body (brain) is a mechanistic notion that thinks of the mind as a gas and the body as a separate container.

Neither our mind, nor our memory, is located inside the body. They are not in the brain, nor in the rest of the body, said Bergson. We have a mind and a memory for the sake of action, and not as a useless luxury. We must consider how they relate to immediate practical action, if we want to understand them.

Where is the mind? Look at your friend doing something like working or thinking. There is the practical mind that exists only in action, in behaviour and in practical thinking during action. Where are your memories of your friend? They exist in your act of recognising this friend. If we sit still, in a total immobilisation of the body and a total inactivation of our mind, then we have no practical mind, nor practical memories anywhere. We don't need them if we don't move around. Practical mind, personality, memory, feelings, and sensitivity are movement-dependent phenomena. We have them for the sake of action, and for no other reason.

Our rational mind is not a practical mind, but a theoretical one, so that it does not operate during action. It is a speculative mind that can only work at rest: this is why we say that we stop to think, and look before we leap. Where the emotional mind is a biological necessity, this rational mind is a human luxury that is not necessary for basic survival.

The theoretical-rational mind examines the world according to theoretical criteria, while the practical-emotional mind assesses the sensory environment on practical grounds alone. An emotional mind is not interested in finding theoretical differences, it makes practical distinctions, only those that are useful for survival. Each mind lives in a different world: one for action, and the other for thinking.

The body is the routine, automated, part of the mind: it is its habitual part that does not change so quickly and easily, because it must perform the repetitive, relatively unvarying, jobs. Nature changes this kind of repetitive movement into a formed structure, because this is engineering that is practical: it is effective and economical. We change our mind more easily than we can change our body and, while changing the body is not impossible, it requires practice: this means constant repetition.

What we now also understand is this: physical matter belongs to physics, it has nothing to do with the difference between body and mind. When we see something, say a ray of light, it is not the same thing that a research scientist in physics will register on his apparatus: a bundle of electromagnetic rays of certain frequencies. It took two thousand million years of progressive evolution to produce that complicated biocomputer we call a human eye that can see light and dark. Light and dark are sensory experiences, they are seen, and not registered as physical waves.

What we ordinarily see is light. Suppose we block that ray of light, so that the room becomes dark. For the scientist this darkness is simply the absence of electromagnetic waves, but for us there is no such thing as seeing an absence. That is impossible. We can never actually see an absence of light, we can understand, but not experience it.

What we see in immediate experience is darkness as some thing that has sensory substance, and is concretely there: a presence. If we feel uneasy at night, such darkness can become a hostile presence, and a threat to our security. For a fearful child, this dark may be a monster that may engulf it to swallow it up. It is not the absence of physical light rays that frightens the child; it is the darkness monster that it sees right there, a thing of some sensory substance.

The child does not experience an absence of physical stimuli, but the presence of an emotional meaning. It is the emotional meaning of the sensory experience that has an impact on our organism, not its physical characteristics. As long as we think of the world as made up of physical matter, we shall not understand its real significance for us as living beings.

It is therefore the emotional meaning of the situation that affects us, and to which we then respond in some way. Sensory material is not physical matter, it is the material of meaning of the world for the organism that lives in it and from it. Whatever we may see, hear, feel, smell, and taste, is always some meaning for action, a practical message for our benefit.

This is to say that a certain situation can have a special meaning that may throw a vulnerable person into despair, while it leaves someone else untouched. The same objective situation has a totally different meaning for this other person, because it is experienced differently. The same apple means different things, and calls up different forms of activity, in a hungry child and an artist who paints it.

A street is a street. One person may walk calmly through it, while another breaks out in a panic, because of a phobia. The same street has a different private emotional meaning for this person, so that she or he may break out into a state of absolute panic over it, while the other is irritated by this phobia: 'For heaven's sake, it is just a street.' Tell that to the child who is frightened by the nightmarish monster of darkness: 'It's just the absence of light', and see how little good that does.

This private part of our experience makes the study of stress difficult. This emotional experience may be only a dim gut reaction, and it is useless to expect a phobic person to say what it is exactly that frightens (assuming a female) her. She does not know that, she only feels it, so that she cannot explain it. How difficult is it to explain a feeling in words? Bear in mind that a picture is worth a thousand words, but that a feeling condenses a thousand pictures: an entire film.

What may be for one personality a traumatic (disorganising) experience, may not be unsettling for another, so we cannot talk about a stress situation without dragging in the personality. We must ask: for whom, for what personality is it traumatic? If we had no personalities, we would have emotional minds that were all the same, duplicates of each other, and we should then experience the world in the same practical-emotional way.

Our personality is a personalised part of a general emotional mind that we all have in common as members of the same human species. Every experience that we have is a general experience for the general emotional mind that we all have in common (we all have feelings that are quite the same), but also a private experience for our personality; these are personal feelings that nobody else may have, and therefore cannot understand adequately.

Psychosomatic medicine is in the process of bringing down the material curtain, and we are now trying to find out how far our emotional mind can influence what goes on in the body, and how we can use this influence to our advantage. This can be done in two ways that are effectively combined: by psychoanalytic intervention, and by means of relaxation and visualisation (e.g. Professor Schultz's autogenic training).

The materialist attitude that is so jealously guarded behind the material curtain is this: there is no evidence to support the claim that situational stress and/or personality factors can represent a significant influence in the natural history of cancer. If there is indeed such an influence, however, then psychiatrists and psychologists would naturally want to become involved in this psychosomatic problem.

The psychosomatic view is that there is enough evidence to support that claim, and that the materialists are simply not willing to admit this. They still think in terms of stale and outdated ideas that exist only behind the material curtain. If there is no evidence to support this claim, or if there is positive evidence to disprove it, then all cancer research and therapy can be strictly limited to oncology and its practical application: oncotherapy.

Once the possibility of emotional influence on the development and progress of cancer has been raised, then it must be looked into because it would be too important to ignore. To illustrate the difficulties in such research, let us take a quick look at what is required. The current investigations move in three (officially five) main directions:

Retrospective studies. This means that the questions about stress are being asked after the cancer has been diagnosed, such as: have you been under stress in the past six months?

There are many things wrong with such an approach:

(a) Who hasn't been stressed in the past six months on looking back, with or without cancer?

(b) When in anger, we can only remember angry things, and when we look back in stress, we can only remember the bad things.

This method is therefore not accurate, but it will give some idea of any major problems in the recent past. It would take many hours of persistent questioning to get a reliable idea of what those six months or so were like.

Prospective studies. Healthy people are studied at random, and from these psychological profiles predictions will be made to see if those that have a cancer-prone personality will indeed develop cancer in the near future. If so, then those claims are right that certain stresses and/or personalities are specifically related to the development of cancer.

Prognostic studies. These are predictions about the outcome of cancer after the diagnosis has been made, and are based on the same psychological considerations. It is clear that cancer treatment can make a mess of such a study, unless a number of different treatment groups are studied:

(i) One group that receives no treatment (almost impossible in practice, unless the patient refuses any form of treatment);

(ii) One group that receives only chemotherapy;

(iii) One group that receives only psychotherapy.

(iv) One group that receives both.

There is a surprising finding everywhere, that many patients who take the opportunity to express their problems, who talk about themselves, who open up about their lives and their fears of the cancer, or who practise relaxation and visualisation in groups or individually, increase their survival significantly.

This, we may assume, is initially (at least) not so much due to an improvement of the biological cancer, but of the mind of the person who has it and wishes to fight it. Mr TCP stops being a TCP, and begins to hope and fight. There should also be little doubt that this can influence the biological cancer, when the regulation systems, especially defence and healing, begin working normally (and that means powerfully) again.

By relaxation and visualisation, it is possible to tap normally unused reserves of regulation that are not needed in a routine practical life. By relaxing, we liberate the emotional mind from its practical task of guiding the body in action, so that we may use it for other, extra-ordinary, purposes. Visualisation for healing is one of them. Practise this method long or short, but practise it consistently.

A SHORT BIBLIOGRAPHY

Bammer, K. & Newberry, B. H., eds.: *Stress and Cancer*, Toronto,
   C. J. Hogreve, 1981.
Bastiaans, J.: *Isolement en bevrijding*, Amsterdam, Uitgeverij
   Balans, 1986.
Bergson, H.: *Matter and memory*, London, George Allen & Unwin
   Ltd, 1970 (original French edition 1896).
   The Creative Mind, New York, Wisdom Library, 1946.
Boss, M.: *"I dreamt last night"*, New York, Gardner Press, 1977.
Brémond, A., Kune, G. A. and Bahnson, C. B.: 'Psychosomatic
   Factors in Breast Cancer Patients'. Elsevier, *Journal of
   Psychosomatic Obstetrics and Gynecology*, 5(1986) 127-136.
Buytendijk, F. J. J.: *Algemene theorie der menselijke houding
   en beweging*, Utrecht, Uitgeverij het Spectrum, 1957.
Cassirer, E.: *The Philosophy of Symbolic Forms*, volume 3,
   New Haven, Yale University Press, 1957.
Dunbar, F.: *Emotions and bodily changes*, New York, Columbia
   University Press, 1949.
Ellenberger, H. F.: *The Discovery of the Unconscious*, New York,
   Basic Books, 1970.
Engel, G.L.: *Psychological development in health and disease*,
   Philadelphia, W.B. Saunders, 1962.
Frank, J. D.: *Persuasion and Healing*, Shocken Books, New York,
   1961.
Freedman, Kaplan, and Sadock, Ed.: *Comprehensive textbook of
   psychiatry*, Baltimore, Williams & Wilkins, 1975.
Greben, S. E.: Rakoff, V. M., Voineskas, G., eds: *A method of
   Psychiatry*, Philadelphia, Lea & Febiger, 1985.
Guex, P.: *An introduction to Psycho-Oncology*, London, Routledge,
   1994.

Hess, W. R.: *The Biology of Mind*, Chicago, University of Chicago Press, 1964.

Heyer, G. R.: *Praktische Seelenheilkunde*, Munich, Ernst Reinhardt Verlag, 1950.

van der Horst, L.: *Anthropologische psychiatrie*, Vol. I, Amsterdam, Van Holkema & Warendorf N.V. 1952.

Janet, P.: *Psychological Healing*, London, George Allen & Unwin, 1925.

Jores, A.: *Der Mensch und seine Krankheit*, Stuttgart, Ernst Kleit Verlag, 1956.

Kroger, W. S.: *Clinical and experimental hypnosis*, Philadelphia, J. B. Lippincott, 1963.

Langen, D. ed.: *Der Weg des Autogenen Trainings*, Darmstadt, Wissenschaftliche Buchgesellschaft, 1976.

van de Loo, K. J. M. ed.: *Psychosomatiek*, Baarn, Uitgeverij Ambo, 1986.

Macfarlane Burnet, F. M., *Self and Not-Self*, Carlton, Melbourne University Press, 1969.

Mack, J. E.: *Nightmares and Human conflict*, Boston, Houghton Mifflin Co, 1974

Menninger, K.: *The Vital Balance*, Hammondsworth, Penguin Books, 1977.

Neher, A.: *The psychology of transcendence*, New Jersey, Prentice Hall, 1980.

Pierpoli, W. & Spector, N. H., Ed.: 'Neuroimmunomodulation: Intervention in Aging and Cancer', *Annals of the New York Academy of Sciences*, vol 521, New York. 1988.

Remplein, H. : *Die Seelische Entwickelung des Menschen im Kindes- und Jugendalter*, Munich, Ernst Reinhardt Verlag, 1958.

Sali, A.: 'Strategies for cancer prevention', *Australian Family Physician* Vol. 16, No. 11, November 1987.

Schultz, J.H.: *Autogenes Training*, Stuttgart, Georg Thieme Verlag, 1979.

Segal. L. & Ron, Y., eds.: *Immunology and Inflammation*, New York. McGraw-Hill Inc, 1994.

Smith, R. T. & Landy, M., eds.: *Immune surveillance*, New York. Academic Press, 1970.

Spiegel, H. and Spiegel, D.: *Trances and Treatment*, Washington, American Psychiatric Press, 1978.

Straus, E.: *Geschehnis und Erlebnis,* Berlin, Springer Verlag, 1978 (reprint of the 1930 edition).
Vom Sinn der Sinne, Berlin, Springer-Verlag, 1978 (Reprint of the 1936 edition).
von Uexküll, Th., ed: *Psychosomatische Medizin,* Munich, Urban & Schwarzenberg, 1986.
Werner, H.: *Comparative Psychology of Mental Development,* New York, Science Editions, 1961.

READING LIST

Dienstfrey. H.: *Where the Mind meets the Body*, New York, Harper Collins Publishers, 1991.

Goleman, D. and Gurim, J.: *Mind Body Medicine*, Marrickville (NSW), A Choice Book, 1995.

Hodgkinson, N.: *Will to be Well*, London, Rider, 1984.

Macfarlane Burnet, F. M., *Self and Not-Self*, Carlton, Melbourne University Press, 1969.

Sali, A.: 'Strategies for cancer prevention', *Australian Family Physician* Vol 16, No. 11, November 1987.

Siegel, B. S.: *Love, Medicine & Miracles*, London, Arrow Books, 1988.

Simonton, O. C., Mathews-Simonton, S., Creighton, J. L.: *Getting Well Again*, Toronto, Bantam Books, 1981.

Shattock, E. H.: *Mind your Body*, London, Thurstone Books, 1979.

Watkins, M. M.: *Waking Dreams*, New York, Interface Book, 1976.